YOUR SKIN & HOW TO LIVE IN IT

YOUR SKIN & HOW TO LIVE IN IT

by Jerome Z. Litt, M.D.

Second Edition

CORINTHIAN PRESS

Publishing Division of EDR Corporation
3592 Lee Road, Shaker Heights, Ohio 44120-5191

Second Edition, First Printing

Printed in the United States of America

Library of Congress Catalog Card No. 81-70956

ISBN 0-86551-016-4

To Vel, without whom....

Acknowledgments

First, to my good friends for their support and encouragement in this enterprise: Dr. Morton A. Shaw, Mr. Fred D. Shapiro, Mr. Saul E. Roth, Dr. Robert W. Fischer, Mr. Joseph T. Zingale, and Mr. Harry Volk.

To the late Dr. Louis Sattler, friend and college mentor; to Mr. Charles Oclassen, friend to all "the healers of the skin"; to Mr. Herb Kamm, for his friendship, for his faith in this venture, and for his help in "turning a phrase"; and to Mr. William Muller, a special friend.

To those dermatologists from whom I learned the science and the art of dermatology: Dr. Harry L. Arnold, Jr., Dr. Rudolf L. Baer, Dr. Benjamin Bender, Dr. Alexander A. Fisher, Dr. Albert M. Kligman, Dr. Morris Leider, the late Dr. Irving L. Schonberg (my former associate), and Dr. Marion B. Sulzberger, genius and *dermatalogue extraordinaire*.

To my dear associate of 18 years, Dr. Harold L. Blumenthal, and to my colleagues—the more than 5,000 dermatologists—with whom I share knowledge, information, and advice.

To my editor, Ms. Linda Jane, for her faith, encouragement, and indispensible help.

To my daughters, Erica, Monica, and Jessica, who have been patient and understanding.

To the more than 78,000 patients who have passed through my office in the past 27 years.

And to that large imposing organ we call SKIN, without which this could not have been written.

Contents

1 Introduction

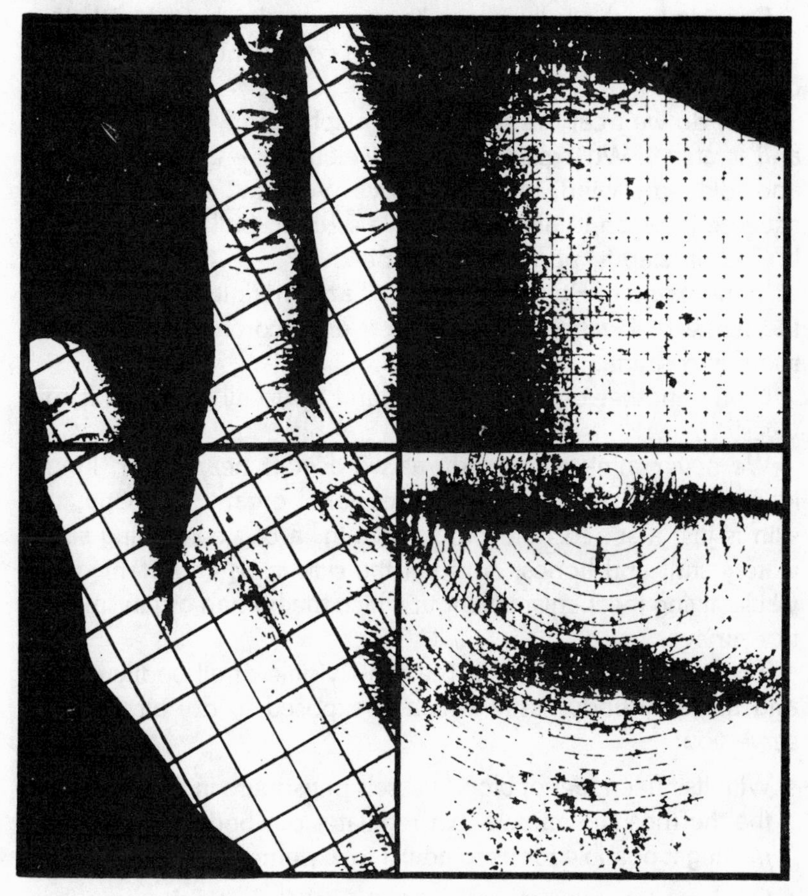

The skin.

Not "skin." *The* skin. The house we live in.

What is this bag we call the skin—this fantastic envelope which possesses some of the most extraordinary mechanisms in the entire body? It is an organ of the body—a marvelously efficient apparatus which nourishes, guards, and protects us 24 hours a day.

When laid out flat, the skin of the average adult would measure some 20 square feet; it would weigh about 9 pounds. That's a lot of organ—one of the largest and heaviest organs of the body.

Also the most abused and maligned organ of the body.

Considering those "thousand natural shocks that [skin] is heir to," its continuing function and lack of complaint is nothing short of amazing.

How do we treat this remarkable mechanism? We dig and rub and scratch it. We expose it to all the elements—extremes of heat and cold, sun, wind, rain, and snow. We cut it, shave it, pick it, squeeze it, pinch it, and twist it. We scrub it, pull it, and bend it. We rub it, slap it, punch it, and knead it.

In the name of Beauty, we paint it and mark it and spray it. In the name of Health, we massage it and scorch it in the steam room and sauna.

Name another organ that can stand up to all that. Yet it survives!

We never think of our skin as we do our heart, liver, lungs, kidneys, brain, or any other "important" organ. To many, the skin is just a sac to hold our insides in, a bag containing some watery stuff and bones. And yet the skin is an important, vital, viable, living mechanism without which the human organism cannot survive.

Think of what your skin, the most visible of all bodily organs and the only body tissue which is exposed to dry air, does to serve you:

- With its fifteen feet of blood vessels per square inch, our skin is the thermostatic miracle that regulates our body temperature, making it possible for us to adjust to extremes of cold and heat.
- Our large integument represents the first line of defense against harmful germs that constantly try to break through and invade our tissues.
- Despite its soft and elastic appearance, our skin is tough enough to withstand a variety of shocks and blows, acting as a cushion to protect the deeper, more vital organs from harm.
- It is a protective barrier between the internal body systems and the hostile environment, which prevents poisonous chem-

icals—liquids and gases—from penetrating the deeper tissues. Recent advances in dermatologic research have shown that our skin helps to metabolize and detoxify certain drugs and potentially dangerous environmental chemicals. At the same time, the skin prevents the outward loss of water, blood, and other essential body fluids. A genuine waterproof sac!

- The skin is our largest organ of sensation, allowing us to perceive heat and cold and various tactile impressions, such as pain. It is the principal organ of communication between us and our environment—the "switchboard" that receives and transmits such information as "the stove is hot," "that knife is sharp," "this pillow is soft."
- It is an organ of excretion, continually eliminating body wastes through more than 2,000,000 sweat pores.
- The skin protects us against the harmful effects of the sun's rays by absorbing them and converting them into dark pigment (tan) to prevent further damage.
- Our skin is supplied with oil glands—100 per square inch—which secrete sebum, the oily material responsible for maintaining the resiliency and elasticity of the skin surface. In addition, this "skin oil" has antibacterial properties which act to destroy various microorganisms that have potential to cause infection.
- Our skin acts as a storage house for water as well as various nutriments, such as sugar and calcium, and helps in the production of Vitamin D.
- Our skin is a mirror of what occurs below the surface—a warning signal of systemic diseases, such as diabetes, shingles, leukemia, and cancer, which often manifest themselves as skin problems long before there is positive evidence of these internal conditions.
- Finally, the skin is endowed with a special capacity to reflect human passions and sentiment. As a mirror of emotions the

skin is without peer. Livid with rage, pale with fright, flushed with pride, blushing with shame. The sweating palm, the anxious pallor. All are release mechanisms of the skin which express combinations of inner feelings and skin reactions to tension, anxiety, and stress.

This, then, is our skin—"the envelope that encloses the letter of our biologic destiny"—the remarkable apparatus that spends a lifetime helping us adjust to our environment. Like a trusted, efficient, uncomplaining housekeeper, it makes life easy for us and protects us from a host of evils. It cleans and washes for us and takes out the garbage. It feeds us, opens the windows, and turns on the heat and air-conditioning. And we take our skin for granted.

What happens when our devoted servant becomes ill? What do we do when we begin to itch? When we develop a rash? Or pimples, blisters, boils, warts, moles, dry skin, flaking and scaling? Pain and burning sensations? Loss of hair? Loss of pigment? Nail problems? Or a host of other signs and symptoms that can plague any portion of our large integument?

What do we do *for* our skin when it rebels? When we develop rashes caused by germs, insects, allergies, internal diseases, hormone imbalance, sun exposure, injuries, and the like?

What do we do for our loyal, trusted, and uncomplaining housekeeper? We become impatient!

"Oh! It's just a simple rash. I'll just smear on a little First Aid Cream or Vitamin A & D Ointment or calamine lotion—or whatever—and it'll probably disappear in a day or two."

Yet it seldom does.

We are not kind to our skin. We abuse it. And although we spend 20 *billion* dollars a year on skin care and cosmetics, we do not understand it. Only when the itching or burning or pain becomes unbearable or when the cosmetic disfigurement becomes embarrassing do we begin to take it seriously.

While the skin is strong and tough, it is also delicate and fragile. The panacea in the jar that promises relief from such diverse conditions as acne, warts, eczema, dry skin, poison ivy dermatitis, diaper rash, and psoriasis is deceptive and misleading. One salve or lotion cannot be beneficial for a dozen different ailments, just as Cinderella's slipper will not fit every foot.

There are over one thousand different diseases and conditions that can affect the skin, hair, and nails. Everyone will, at one time or another, develop some type of problem that deals with this large integumentary system. Everyone....

Warts, dandruff, dry skin, moles, athlete's foot. Excess hair or not enough hair. Rashes from the sun, from germs, from poison ivy. Insects bites, cold sores, hives, rectal itch. Wrinkles, large pores, stretch marks or scars.

Job had boils.

Caesar was bald. Queen Elizabeth I lost every hair on her body.

Napoleon had scabies.

Tolstoy had canker sores. Wagner had eczema.

Ernest Hemingway had psoriasis.

Winston Churchill had a persistent, intolerable, dry skin itch.

Dr. Tom Dooley had a melanoma and died from it.

Lyndon B. Johnson had skin cancer.

Golda Meir had shingles.

Telly Savalas has a mole. So does Elizabeth Taylor.

Tens of millions of people all over the world have acne, warts and eczema.

Your male friends may have hair loss, athlete's foot, or jock itch; your female friends may complain of large pores, stretch marks, and "zits." And almost all adult women have cellulite!

Your children will have impetigo, diaper rash, ringworm, acne, warts, cradle cap, birthmarks, and insect bites.

Your parents will develop dry skin, wrinkles, skin tumors, leg ulcers, and shingles.

And how many of you are plagued with canker sores? Rectal itch? What about the eight million Americans who have psoriasis? And the countless millions who are frustrated by eczema?

No one can escape.

What This Book Can Do for You

In the following pages you'll learn about a few dozen conditions that commonly affect the skin and hair. Many of them are not diseases in the sense that they cause some bodily dysfunction, but they are important enough to affect the general well-being and psychological health of those afflicted. You'll learn something about the causes and symptoms of these disorders and the different methods doctors use to treat them.

After many of the chapters, you'll find sections describing what you yourself can do to prevent, manage, or eliminate particular skin conditions. Please understand that there is no magic in the treatment of skin disease. The skin, like every other organ, can develop "instant" maladies—maladies which may take weeks or months to heal or cure. The sunburn that develops in an hour, the cold sores or poison ivy dermatitis that can begin overnight, the pimples or boils that erupt in a day, the hives that develop in minutes from aspirin or penicillin—all may take days or weeks of constant medication to get them under control.

The products which I mention in these treatment sections are known as "over-the-counter" (o-t-c) medications which you can purchase at your local drugstore without a doctor's prescription. Some of these are oral medications, medications that you take by mouth. Others are "topical," or local, medications that you apply directly on the area you're treating.

Many of the preparations require that a pharmacist "mix and make" them for you. This is known as "compounding." Your pharmacist may be reluctant to compound a preparation for you. Compounding is time-consuming, exacting, and sometimes messy. It is much easier for the pharmacist to take a tube or a jar from the shelf, remove the existing label, and affix the pharmacy's own label with the required directions. Understandably, your pharmacist will charge for the time it takes to make up your "special" batch, but in the long run compounded preparations are more economical.

When using any medication, follow the directions on the label or the directions I have provided. Be careful to note any special precautions. You must realize that all people do not respond alike to every medication—local, oral, or by injection. The salve that's so beneficial for Portia might cause Stevie to break out. The soothing lotion for Herb might cause burning on Fred's skin. And there are some people who, unfortunately, develop an allergy (sensitivity) to almost every kind of topical medication.

If you find that a preparation causes some unpleasant symptom, such as burning, stinging, pain, or increased itching, discontinue it at once. It could be that you are—or have become—allergic to one or more of the ingredients in it. If this occurs, try a different type or brand of medication.

While I have mentioned dozens of products for the management of over forty skin ailments, there are literally hundreds of others that may serve the same purposes. The products I have listed are ones that I personally prescribe and recommend in my private practice of dermatology—a practice that numbers well over 78,000 patients. I have tested these products over the years, and while I cannot speak for *all* the other 5,000 dermatologists in this country, a majority of them recommend the same preparations.

Lastly, do not hesitate to see your physician. This book is *not* intended to replace his or her expertise. Rather, it is intended to help you better understand your skin and how to live in it.

2 Dermatologic Dozen

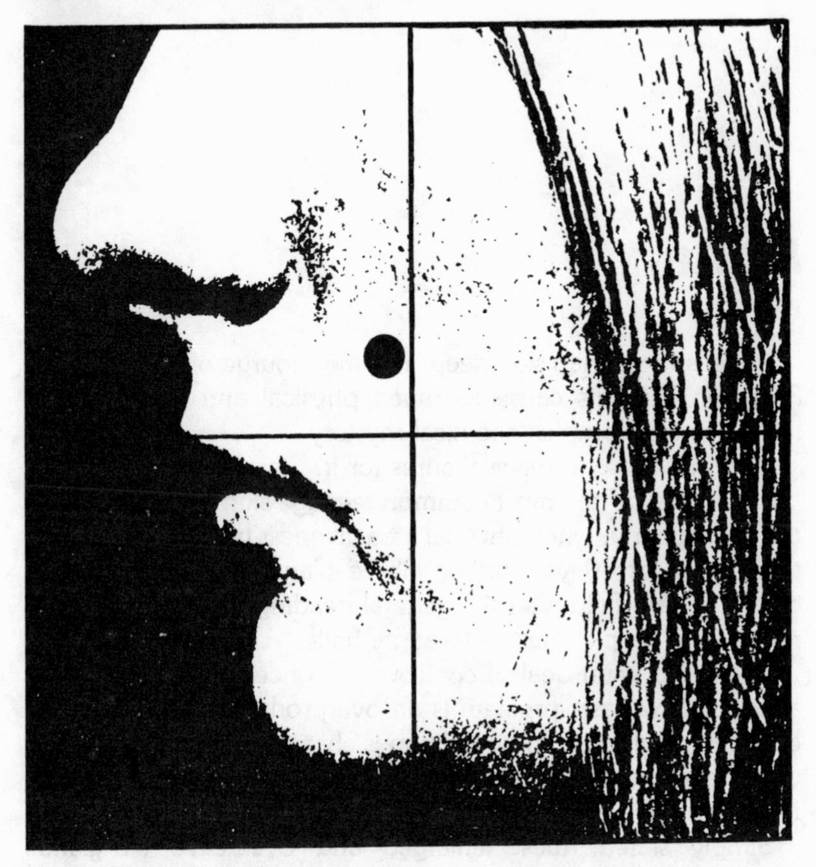

There are some skin diseases which are much more common than others. Acne, for example, will occur in nine out of ten youngsters, making it the most common skin ailment seen by the dermatologist—the specialist in medicine who is trained in diseases of the skin.

This chapter deals with the twelve most common dermatologic complaints—what I refer to as the Dermatologic Dozen. These occur with sufficient frequency to comprise at least 90% of a dermatologist's office practice.

Acne

Acne is more than skin deep. It is the scourge of adolescence. Few skin ailments cause as much physical and psychological misery as this complex chemical mystery.

And there are no magical cures for it.

Acne is by far the most common teenage skin disorder. At the onset of puberty, when physical attractiveness becomes so important, 9 out of 10 youngsters will be plagued by the unsightly blemishes that fall under the general heading of acne. They can range from simple pimples to angry boils.

There is a great deal of controversy concerning the "why" of acne, but the basic problem is an overproduction of skin oil by enlarged oil glands. This condition is characteristic of the internal chemical changes that occur at puberty when the skin is adjusting to a greatly increased output of hormones.

Simply stated, these enlarged and overactive oil glands become clogged, forming blackheads and whiteheads. The glands continue to manufacture oil which cannot escape.

Bacteria, which naturally reside on the skin in "friendly" numbers, begin to thrive in these trapped secretions and become "unfriendly," causing infected pimples. These may lead to cysts, which then break down to form scars.

Acne occurs on areas of the body where oil glands are the largest, most numerous, and most active: the face, chest, and back.

Many factors can aggravate acne. Anything that prevents the oily secretions from flowing freely out of the oversized oil gland, such as infrequent cleansing, long hair (particularly bangs), greasy hair dressings, so-called moisturizers, and other cosmetics containing lanolin, will further plug up the already clogged oil gland opening to produce new lesions.

Youngsters working around filling stations and fast food restaurants, who are constantly exposed to greases and oils, are especially prone to acne flare-ups.

Hormonal disorders, as well as drugs such as cortisone, iodides, and anti-epilepsy medications, also can aggravate acne. Young women often experience an acne eruption just before their menstrual period. The "low-dose" birth control pills also are responsible for acne in women who never had the problem as adolescents. There also is some indication that acne around the mouth is aggravated by fluoridated toothpaste.

Acne usually lasts for several years and abates in the early 20s. The conflicts and tensions that may arise along the way can lead to feelings of inferiority, insecurity, and inadequacy which undermine self-confidence. After acne has burned itself out, it may leave permanent scars on the psyche as well as on the skin. Both subside with time, but if the skin scars are severe, they may benefit from further treatment.

Every day brings promise of a new magical cure. The latest heralded treatment for acne—at least two years away from commercial distribution—is an oral drug of the Vitamin A family, 13-*cis*-retinoic acid. This new treatment is said to be highly effective for the severe, scarring, antibiotic-resistant form of cystic acne known as acne conglobata. However, it is not thought to be effective for the common, garden-variety type of everyday acne.

While there is no easy cure for acne, it can be controlled to lessen its severity and to prevent the pitting and scarring that arise from neglect and self-medication.

Don't be discouraged if progress is slow. If you are diligent, conscientious, and faithful with your treatment, you will reap the benefit of a clear complexion.

It is especially important that parents try to understand their teenagers' plight. By offering encouragement and helping your teenager maintain his or her self-esteem, you can help lessen the mental anguish and psychological scars that so often accompany acne.

Here are a few general principles that can help prevent or control acne:

- Wash thoroughly at least three times daily.
- Don't pick or squeeze.
- Shampoo frequently.
- Keep hair off the face and don't use greasy hair dressings.
- Discontinue your fluoridated toothpaste for a few months if you have acne near your mouth and note whether it makes any difference.
- Avoid greasy cosmetics and hair sprays.
- Avoid emotional stress.

The role that diet plays in causing acne is controversial and debatable. I recommend restricting chocolate, seafood, nuts, and sharp cheese and limiting milk intake to three glasses a day.

If your physician has prescribed tetracycline for your acne, do not take multiple-vitamin supplements containing iron. Iron interferes with the absorption of tetracycline.

If your acne is stubborn, persistent, and disfiguring, consult your physician. Acne can result in permanent scarring if left untreated. Your physician can prescribe internal and topical medications to eliminate or lighten this cross that almost all youngsters have to bear.

Treating Acne

The following is a list of some of the specific measures and products I recommend to reduce, eliminate, or "mask" acne lesions. There are countless products available for controlling acne, and new products are being developed all the time. I have limited this list to those products that give my patients best results.

Soaps & Cleansers

Wash your face thoroughly at least three times daily. For mild acne, where there are mainly blackheads and some oiliness, use:

Acnaveen Soap (Cooper)
Fostex Cake (Westwood)
Neutrogena Acne Soap (Neutrogena)

For the more severe type of acne, when you need extra degreasing, try a good abradant cleanser:

Pernox Scrub (Westwood)
Ionax Scrub (Owen)
PanOxyl Bar (Stiefel)

Shampoos

Shampoo daily. Patients with acne usually have oily hair. When too much oil collects on the scalp and hair, it manages to get on the skin, further plugging up the already clogged oil glands. An interesting phenomenon is that girls (and boys) with unusually long hair—no matter how they style it—very often have acne on their backs.

For exceptionally oily hair, use one of the following:

Pernox Shampoo (Westwood)
Soltex Shampoo (C&M Pharmacal)
Ionil Shampoo (Owen)

Keep your hair off your face, eliminate bangs, and avoid hair sprays and greasy hair dressings. Use creme rinses in moderation.

Lotions, Creams, & Gels

For mild cases of acne, apply any of the following lotions or gels to the affected pimples once or twice daily:

Acne-Aid Lotion (tinted or clear) (Stiefel)
Fostril Lotion (Westwood)
Komed Lotion (mild) (Barnes-Hind)
Transact Gel (Westwood)
Neutrogena Acne Drying Gel (Neutrogena)

For moderate to severe acne, where there are many blackheads and "zits," you may want to try one of the following lotions. They all contain benzoyl peroxide, a very effective medication for the more stubborn cases of acne. These medications are often recommended by dermatologists.

Benoxyl 5 Lotion (Stiefel)
Vanoxide Lotion (Dermik)
Persadox Lotion 5% (Owen)

These preparations should cause slight peeling to help dry up your zits. If your face gets too dry, use the products less often.

If your face begins to itch, burn, or turn red from using any of these preparations, you may be allergic to one of the ingredients. Stop the medication at once and apply cool, wet compresses to your face. Do not use the medication again. Use a different or a milder preparation.

For more stubborn acne problems (if no peeling develops from the use of any of the above) try one of the following:

Benoxyl 10 Lotion (Stiefel)
Persadox HP Cream or **Lotion** (Owen)
Fostex BPO Anti Bacterial Acne Gel (Westwood)

Other Acne Aids

Degreasing Liquids (follow directions on the package):

Drytex (C & M Pharmacal)
Ionax Astringent Cleanser (Owen)
Seba-Nil Liquid Cleanser (Owen)

Degreasing Pads (follow directions on the package):

Seba-Nil Towelettes (Owen)
Stri-Dex Pads (Lehn & Fink)

"Therapeutic" Make-ups and Cover-ups:

Liquimat Lotion (Owen)
Clearasil Regular Tinted Cream (Vick Chemical)
Acnotex Lotion (C & M Pharmacal)

Cosmetics

Avoid greasy cosmetics. An oil-free, water-based cosmetic cover-up is the best type of make-up even for those who do *not* have acne problems.

Make-ups best suited for acne skin are liquids which can be easily shaken in the bottle. The thicker make-ups, those in a tube or jar or cake or stick, usually contain greases or oils which plug up the already clogged oil glands.

Don't be misled by deceptive labeling, such as: "dermatologist-tested," "pH-balanced," "hypo-allergenic," and "natural." These are meaningless terms which only lure unsuspecting buyers into believing they are getting something special. All you should demand is "oil-free" and "water-based." The rest is gimmickry.

A few of the better cover-ups, those less likely to aggravate or cause acne, are:

Clinique: Pore Minimizer
Revlon: Touch and Glow
Estée Lauder: Fresh Air
Ultima: Skim Milk
Revlon: Moon Drops

In addition, Almay, Ar-Ex, Marcelle, and Owen Laboratories (Allercreme) all manufacture a whole line of oil-free make-ups for acne patients. Try one; try all. Only you can decide what's best for you.

Moisturizers

Finally, if you need a moisturizer, the only acceptable ones that I recommend are the following:

Aquaderm (C & M Pharmacal)
Wibi Dry Skin Lotion (Owen)
T&C Therapeutic Cream (unscented) (Dermalab)

Note: If you have acne on one cheek only or more on one cheek, you may have the habit of resting that cheek on your palm. Try to break the habit and wear a white cotton glove on that hand when you go to bed at night.

Warts

Warts are benign tumors of the skin caused by specific viruses. They *never* become cancerous.

But while warts usually are perfectly harmless, they should be destroyed because they are infectious, unsightly, and occasionally painful.

Warts can be passed on to others by direct or indirect contact, in such places as locker rooms, public shower stalls, gymnasium mats and swimming pools. They also can spread on the same individual by picking, scratching, shaving, or biting one's nails.

There are various types of warts, depending upon their location and their form or configuration.

The so-called common, or vulgar, warts are raised, rough-textured, grayish-looking, painless growths which can vary in size from that of a pinhead to a fairly large mass. While they may occur on any portion of the skin surface, common warts usually are found on the fingers, hands, and the soles of the feet.

The flat (or plane) warts, appearing as smooth, flesh-colored, slightly elevated, matchhead-sized lesions, occur chiefly on the face and backs of the hands of children and young adults.

Genital warts are found in the moist areas of the genital and anal regions.

Warts on the sole are known as plantar warts. (Not "planter's warts," as some people are fond of saying, as if there were something agricultural or occupational about them.) These warts are the most stubborn variety and frequently resist all known treatments.

The fact that there are dozens of widely proclaimed plans for eliminating warts attests to the fact that there is no single predictably effective agent or method. Ideally, the treatment for warts should be quick, safe, painless and should produce no unsightly or lasting scars.

Folklore Remedies for Warts

Rub warts with a raw potato, then bury the potato in clay. Just to be on the safe side, repeat with another potato the next day.

Rub warts with a black snail and impale the snail on a thorn tree. When the snail dries and withers, so do the warts.

Rub warts with a cinder, tie the cinder up in paper, and leave it at a crossroads. Whoever picks up the parcel and unwraps it, catches the warts.

Prick the wart with a gooseberry thorn passed through a wedding ring.

Lick your forefinger and point it at a passing funeral three times and say,"My warts go with you."

Rub the wart with a piece of stolen beef. Then bury the meat.

Take a dead black cat to a graveyard at midnight. When you hear a noise, throw the cat toward the sound. That will take the warts away.

Steal a greasy dishrag from your neighbor. Wipe your warts with it, then throw it over your left shoulder into a pond.

Some physicians recommend that the best way to manage warts is to let them manage themselves. If left untreated, half of all the warts people are afflicted with (and there are 20 million people in this country with warts) will disappear in about two years.

This seems to be the natural history of warts.

Warty people, however, do not want to wait for any spontaneous cure, and so they seek out medical advice.

Methods physicians use to treat warts are about as varied as warts themselves. The type of treatment depends upon many factors, including your age, the location of the warts, and the size and number of warts to be treated.

A physician may use electrosurgery, in which the wart is burned off with an electric needle under local anesthesia. There is also chemical destruction (which uses various types of acids, plasters, and other chemicals). Other warts are frozen off, using liquid nitrogen at minus 320 degrees Fahrenheit, or dry ice. Some warts succumb to surgical excision (cutting the wart out under local anesthesia). A less-widely used method is X-ray therapy carefully administered by a dermatologist or radiologist. In selected cases this type of therapy can produce miracles, but the recent concern over the effects of radiation has restricted its use.

Some physicians (and some grandmothers) charm warts away by suggestive methods. These "witching" methods have worked in many individuals, particularly young, impressionable children and they leave no scars, no matter how deep or long-standing the warts may have been. Regardless of how bizarre or ludicrous a treatment may sound, if the patient has faith in the "charmer," the warts usually will disappear. (However, I do not recommend stealing a piece of beef or a dishrag!)

A great deal of research is going on to determine why certain people get warts, why others do not, and why warts sometimes disappear spontaneously. In the meantime, if you can't ward off warts, take comfort in knowing that your doctor can help get rid of them.

Treating Warts

Local Medications

For the small, flat warts that usually appear on the face and the backs of the hands (especially in children) ask your pharmacist for the following:

Castor Oil (1-oz. bottle)

Directions: Apply the castor oil to the warts twice daily, using a cotton-tipped applicator (Q-Tip).

For the common, "vulgar" warts located over the fingers, palms, feet, and other areas, use either:

Compound W Wart Remover (Whitehall)

Directions: Apply to the warts at night. Do not cover.

Wart-Away (DePree)

Directions: Same as above.

Or ask your pharmacist to compound my favorite wart "recipe" in an applicator bottle (this has a glass rod to apply the medication):

Salicylic acid	**10%**
Lactic acid	**10%**
Flexible Collodion	**to make ½ oz.**

Directions: Apply to the warts at night.

"Exorcism"

For stubborn warts around and under the fingernails, use the following method which I "invented." I call it "adhesotherapy."

Completely wrap the wart with four layers of plain adhesive tape. (See diagram for instructions on wrapping the tape.) Do not wrap too tightly! Leave on for six and one-half days. Remove for half a day. Repeat the entire procedure (6½ days on, ½ day off). After three or four weeks of this regimen, the wart "gets tired" and disappears, leaving no scar.

Note: When treating children's warts in this manner, just before the "ears" are snipped off, parents can draw a "happy" face (2). The children will appreciate your sense of humor, take you into their confidence, and the warts will disappear even faster!

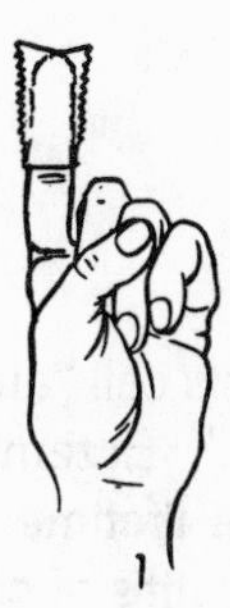

1

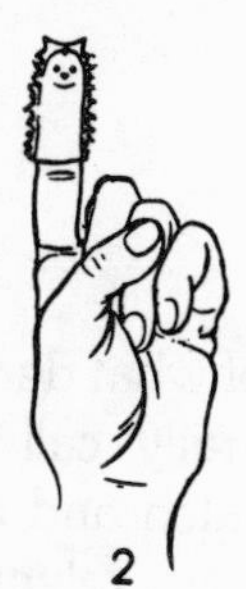

2

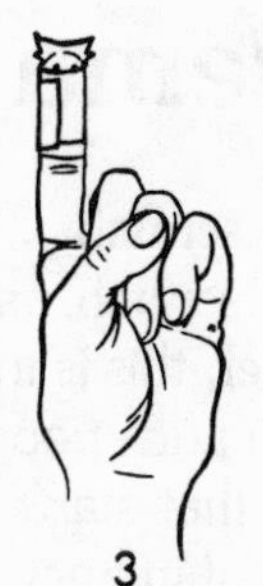

3

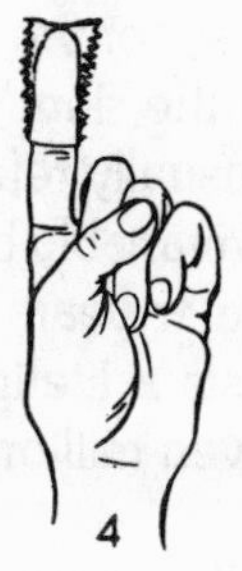

4

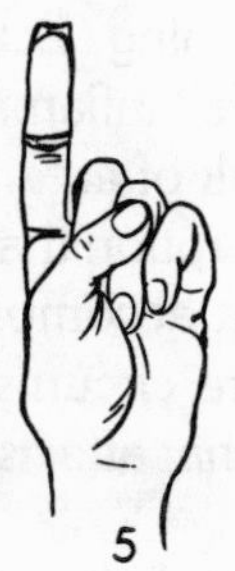

5

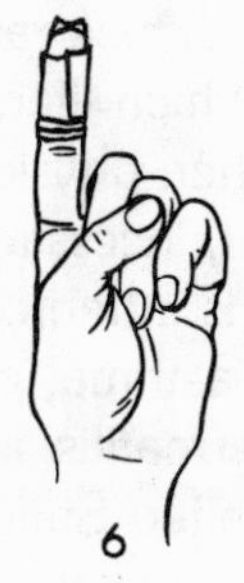

6

Eczema

Itch...scratch...

Itch...scratch...scratch...

In brief, this is the story of what dermatologists call "atopic dermatitis" and people generally call "eczema." Eczema is the disease that starts from scratch and may last a lifetime. It is the eczema of infancy, the chronic, relentless dermatitis of childhood and adolescence, and the fierce and uncontrollable itching of the adult.

What do we mean by eczema?

Eczema is a non-specific, general term which, to most people, means a diffuse rash with itching. Eczema is a synonym for dermatitis, which literally means "inflammation of the skin."

But when physicians speak of eczema, they usually refer to the persistent, incessant itchy eruption that almost invariably begins in infancy, is inherited, is often accompanied in later years by hayfever or asthma, and in rare circumstances lasts a lifetime. It is atopic dermatitis, a disease that affects about seven million people in the United States alone.

No one as yet knows the "why" of this virtually uncontrollable, allergic process. It begins entirely with itching on a perfectly normal-looking skin. You then scratch where it itches and you yourself produce the dermatitis we know of as eczema.

There are three different "stages" of atopic dermatitis:

1. The *infantile form* ("infantile eczema"). This usually begins about 6 or 8 weeks after birth. (Interestingly enough, the newborn is usually free of this condition.) The itching at this age—and up until the age of two years—is often intense. The rash usually worsens after vaccinations and immunization injections and during the teething phase.

2. *The childhood type.* While the infantile form in over half the cases fades out between the ages of two and four, it may continue on into the so-called childhood type of eczema. This later stage, however, may develop without any prior infantile eczema. The areas that suffer most in this type of eczema are the creases in the elbows and the bends of the knees. The affected areas are more dry and the skin becomes thickened and grayish in color. The itching becomes fierce, and the children are restless, anxious, and hyperactive.

3. *The adolescent and adult types.* In many cases the infantile and childhood eczemas disappear after a few years only to reappear in late adolescence. While it usually fades away by the age of 30, it may persist throughout the entire lifetime of some unfortunate person. The itching, as before, may be intense and is usually worse at night. The areas affected are the bends of the elbows and knees, the face, the shoulders, and the upper back. The itchy and scratched skin becomes thickened and heavily pigmented and develops dry scales.

There is no specific or uniform treatment for this torment since the areas affected and the degree of itching affect different people in different ways. At best, we can attempt to alleviate the fierce itching which, in essence, *is* the disease. Interrupt and terminate this fearful symptom and we break the itch-scratch reflex which is wholly responsible for the clinical manifestation—the rash.

Although there is no specific treatment for controlling eczema, there are some general rules and measures:

- Never use soap! Soap removes the natural oils from the already overdry skin. Use soap substitutes, such as Lowila Cake or Aveenobar, for all cleansing purposes.
- Take baths and showers in lukewarm—not hot—water. Add soothing bath oils to the water for excessively dry, scaly skin.
- Avoid sudden extremes of temperature and any violent exercise that causes sweating. Going from a hot to a cold or from a cold to a hot environment will trigger the itching mechanism.
- Eliminate fuzzy, rough, and woolen clothing as these aggravate eczema. Soft, loose, cotton clothing is best.
- Get rid of furry and fuzzy toys and feather pillows.
- And, while it may seem cruel to some families, removing household pets, particularly long-haired cats and dogs, is a must.
- Do not work around dust, industrial chemicals, fumes, sprays, cutting oils, and solvents. All these tend to aggravate eczema.
- Avoid all cosmetics, cleansers, body oils, and lotions that contain lanolin. Lanolin is good for sheep but bad for humans. It causes allergies, plugs up oil glands (causing acne), and aggravates eczema. Besides, would you apply to your skin a substance that is advertised as being great for polishing shoes and cleaning pots?
- Don't wear rubber gloves for household chores. Even the cotton-lined varieties tend to "sweat" when immersed in hot water and thereby leach out the chemicals and stabilizers in the rubber which only aggravate eczema skin of the fingers and hands. If you find that you must do the housework and dishes with rubber gloves, get cotton liners (Dermal Gloves) and wear them at all times under the rubber gloves.
- Avoid colds and other upper respiratory infections which tend to lower the resistance of the skin and aggravate atopic dermatitis.

- Never expose yourself to people who have cold sores (fever blisters) or who have recently had smallpox vaccinations. The viruses that cause cold sores and smallpox can cause serious and sometimes fatal eruptions in those who have eczema.
- Avoid over-the-counter salves and lotions, particularly those containing benzocaine and antibiotics.
- Do not use Vaseline and other occlusive greasy ointments. These tend to aggravate the itching by preventing the evaporation of sweat.
- During the winter holidays, avoid real Christmas trees. The artificial varieties are less irritating and less allergenic to eczema sufferers.
- Whenever possible, avoid emotional stress and tension. There is no other skin condition—psoriasis, acne, lichen planus, etc.—where "nerves" play a greater role.

If the rash persists and the itching is uncontrollable, see your general doctor or pediatrician. He or she will be able to prescribe those time-tested remedies in the form of creams and lotions, and, where necessary, "relatives" of cortisone and, perhaps, antibiotics, if the rash becomes infected.

Treating Acute Eczema

For the acute, weeping, and oozing type of eczema, soothing wet dressings and baths can help relieve the inflammation and itching.

Compresses

For the localized, acute eczemas, use either of the following:

Domeboro Powder Packets (Dome)

Directions: Dissolve contents of one packet in a pint (16 oz.) of warm water and apply as open wet dressings (see page 208 for directions on how to apply wet dressings). Use for 15 or 20 minutes every 2 or 3 hours.

Bluboro Powder (Herbert)

Directions: Same as above.

Baths

For the widespread or extensive cases of acute eczema, the best form of therapy is a soothing bath taken in any of the following:

Aveeno Colloidal Oatmeal (Cooper)

Directions: See directions on the container.

Alpha Keri Therapeutic Bath Oil (Westwood)

Directions: Add 2 to 4 capfuls to a half tub of warm water. Soak for 20 to 30 minutes once or twice daily.

nutraSpa Bath Oil (Owen)

Directions: Same as above.

Treating Subacute Eczema

Creams & Lotions

When the weeping and oozing have begun to dry up, discontinue the wet dressings. Now you can use a cream to help relieve the itching and permit the skin to maintain its smoothness and resiliency. Have your pharmacist make up the following:

Menthol	**¼%**
Phenol	**½%**
Cold Cream	**to make 4 oz.**

Directions: Apply every 3 or 4 hours and after bath.

(*Caution*: Never use preparations containing phenol over widespread areas of the body, and never use them in infants.)

Or use the following o-t-c creams or lotions:

Rhulicort Cream (Lederle)
Rhulicort Lotion (Lederle)
Schamberg's Lotion (C & M Pharmacal)
Directions: Same as above.

Treating Chronic Eczema

Lubricating Preparations

For the dry, scaly chronic variety of eczema, where the skin is tight and thickened, you may want to try lubricating preparations. For localized patches of chronic, dry eczema, try the following compounded preparation:

Menthol	**¼%**
Phenol	**½%**
Eucerin Emulsion	**to make 4 oz.**

Directions: Apply 2 or 3 times daily. Also, see caution above.

Or try the following o-t-c preparation:

Vioform Ointment 3% (Ciba)

Directions: Apply 2 or 3 times daily. (*Note:* This preparation may stain clothing and skin.)

Baths

For generalized, chronic eczema, baths using the following bath additives may be helpful in relieving the itching and in softening the skin:

Aveeno Oilated (Cooper)
Directions: Follow the directions on the container.

Balnetar (Westwood)
Directions: 2 to 4 capfuls to a tub of warm water and soak for 20-30 minutes daily.

Shampoo

T/Gel Shampoo (Neutrogena)

Treating All Stages of Eczema

Soap Substitutes

Never use soaps. Use either of the following soap substitutes for all cleansing purposes:

Lowila Cake (Westwood)
Aveenobar (Cooper)

Oral Medications

For the itching that accompanies virtually all eczema, take any of the following antihistamines every 4 hours when necessary. (See directions and cautions on the label for proper dosage.)

Chlor-Trimeton Tablets 4 mg (Schering)
Chlor-Trimeton Syrup (Schering)
Dimetane Tablets 4 mg (Robins)

Note: Never use topical medications containing:

- "-caine" derivatives, the most common being benzocaine.
- antihistamine creams and lotions, such as Caladryl, Ziradryl, Surfadil, and Calamox.

Psoriasis

Psoriasis is a stubborn, chronic, and as yet incurable disease of the skin. Some eight million people suffer from psoriasis in the United States alone. And they spend more than one billion dollars a year ($2000 every minute!) to treat this poorly understood ailment.

Psoriasis, the "disease of healthy people," doesn't threaten or shorten the lives of those who are afflicted with it. It is neither an infection nor an allergy. It probably is not due to any vitamin or mineral deficiency. It doesn't leave scars or make you lose your hair. In fact, it may not even itch. To the psoriasis sufferer, however, it can be an emotionally traumatic disorder.

Psoriasis is characterized by patches of raised, red skin covered by silvery-white scales. It can occur at any age, commonly beginning in young adulthood, and usually recurs at unpredictable intervals. It may be worse in the winter and is often precipitated or aggravated by physical or emotional stress, upper respiratory infections, strep throat, and skin injuries.

Psoriasis is not contagious. It does seem to run in families, although the pattern of heredity is not clear.

No one knows the cause of psoriasis, but we do know how it comes about. Normal skin cells have a life span of about 28 days. This is the time it takes for a cell to be born, move to the outer surface of the skin, and flake off.

In psoriasis, the skin cells turn over at a rate 10 times faster than the normal cells, causing a build-up of scales in thick, red, and sharply-bordered patches. These patches may be small—the size of a matchhead or smaller—or extremely large—covering the entire body. If these patches occur in the body's creases and folds, they may cause itching and pain. Although any part of the skin may be affected, the patches usually occur on the elbows, knees, and scalp.

Psoriasis comes in many shapes and forms. It can, for example, be limited to the fingernails and toenails in the form of small pits or stippling. In some unfortunate people, it affects the genital area and can limit sexual activity. In extreme cases, it is widespread, causing severe embarrassment which, in turn, can lead to psychological problems: the true "heartbreak" of psoriasis.

If you have psoriasis, there are some remedies you can try yourself. But for serious or stubborn cases, I recommend you see your physician. There are many treatments, both new and old, which require a doctor's expertise.

The method of treatment depends on the extent and severity of the symptoms. An old standby is one of the various types of tar preparations which have been used with good results by thousands of psoriasis sufferers. Other methods are sunlight, ultraviolet radiation, and X-ray therapy. There are also cortisone-like preparations that are applied to or injected into the patches and various oral medications which, while often effective, may have potentially serious side effects. Make sure your doctor explains the possible side effects before you enter into any treatment.

Every new treatment for psoriasis becomes headline news. Most of these "miracle treatments" quickly fall into disfavor or are discarded when another "breakthrough" is heralded. The latest magical cure for psoriasis is called the PUVA treatment. The person swallows a harmless drug called methoxsalen and then is exposed to longwave ultraviolet light. The proponents of this new type of treatment swear by it, and today it has become the most fashionable therapy for those afflicted with extensive or generalized psoriasis. There is some indication, however, that this treatment can lead to severe skin damage appearing many years later. Another newly-reported treatment is bathing in the Dead Sea!

But let's face it...while many of these treatments can help relieve the itching and scaling, there is no known "cure" for psoriasis. The cure will come about only when we know the exact nature and mechanism of the disease.

For now, the psoriasis sufferer can take comfort in the fact that, with the variety of medications and treatments available, this potentially traumatic and hopeless disorder has a good chance of being controlled.

Treating Psoriasis

There is no reliable, sure-fire treatment for psoriasis, but you can often relieve the scaling and the itching that accompany this condition.

Baths

For generalized or widespread psoriatic patches, tar baths are very helpful, provided you are not allergic to tar. Try one of the following tar preparations in your bath. Directions for each are on the bottle.

Balnetar (Westwood)
Lavatar (Doak)
Polytar Bath Oil (Stiefel)

Soaps

In addition to the bath, you may want to try a soap which can help in reducing extensive psoriatic scaling:

Polytar Soap (Stiefel)
Packer's Pine Tar Soap (Cooper)

Local Medications

Various types of tar medicaments—alone or in combination—can be very effective in controlling localized patches of psoriasis. They are safer and less expensive than the cortisone-type medications your doctor may prescribe. However, they all stink, sting, and stain. The following are some of the more popular and effective creams, ointments, and gels containing tar:

Estar Gel (Westwood)
psoriGel (Owen)
Alphosyl Cream (Reed & Carnrick)
Pragmatar (SKF)
Tegrin (Block)
Mazon (Thayer)

Note: Never apply these to inflamed skin and avoid contact with the eyes. In rare instances, any of the above may cause some type of allergic sensitivity.

An inexpensive, vanishing-type preparation that often gives good results can be made up by your pharmacist:

Salicylic acid	**3%**
Cold Cream	**to make 4 oz.**

Directions: Apply to the affected areas twice daily.

Shampoos

For psoriasis of the scalp, one of the most stubborn areas of the body to treat, it is important to shampoo often (daily or twice daily!) and thoroughly. Some of the better and more effective shampoos include those with tar. Try them all and see which is best for you.

T/Gel (Neutrogena) (no tar odor)
Polytar (Stiefel) (doesn't stain hair)
Pentrax (Cooper)
Sebutone (Westwood)
Zetar (Dermik)
DHS Tar (Persōn & Covey)
Ionil T (Owen)

After-Shampoo Treatment

If your scalp condition is stubborn, use the following lotion:

Neomark Lotion (C & M Pharmacal)

Directions: Rub into scalp at night using a cotton ball.

Oral Medication

If your psoriasis itches, take the following antihistamine every four hours. It may cause drowsiness, so read the label for dosage and warnings.

Chlor-Trimeton Tablets 4 mg (Schering)

Sunlight

About 85% of people with psoriasis benefit from sunlight. About 15% either get worse or are not affected at all by exposure to the sun. If the sun does help, it sometimes pays to invest in a good hot quartz sunlamp (Hanovia). When carefully used according to the manufacturer's or physician's instructions, this machine will relieve many a psoriasis sufferer.

Diet

Some people benefit from restricting certain foods. Several patients of mine are made worse after eating seafood; some after drinking liquor or beer. Some drugs, taken internally, such as lithium, also aggravate psoriasis. If you think something is making your psoriasis worse, try to be a detective and eliminate the culprit.

Cold Sores and Genital Herpes

Like the common cold, cold sores of the oral and genital regions are frequent, worldwide, and unresponsive to present-day treatments. They are also highly contagious, which, particularly in the case of genital herpes, can be very distressing.

The typical cold sore consists of a small group of water blisters on a reddened base. This blister group may itch, prickle, or burn and can vary in size from that of a matchhead to a 25-cent piece or ever larger. Although a cold sore can develop on any part of the body, it generally occurs on the mouth, the lips, or the genital areas.

Up until a few years ago, it was thought that cold sores of the mouth and lips—transmitted by contact with infected saliva—were invariably caused by a virus called herpesvirus Type 1. And that cold-sore-like infections below the waist—genital herpes—were always caused by a closely-related organism, labelled herpesvirus Type 2. In recent years, however, due perhaps to our changing mores and the growing popularity of oral sex, the Type 1 herpesvirus can cause genital "cold sores" and the Type 2 herpesvirus can cause mouth and lip lesions.

Cold Sores of the Mouth and Lips

Whether you call them cold sores, fever blisters, or the medical term herpes simplex, they all describe the same problem—a problem that literally can lead to a pain in the neck.

The primary, or initial, infection with the herpes simplex virus usually occurs in early childhood. However, the infection may not become evident for a long time (even 30 years!) while the virus lies dormant. Although highly contagious, these infections generally are of a benign nature and are more irritating than they are dangerous.

The visible sign of the infection, the blisters, can be triggered by such diverse forces as sun exposure, local trauma (from dental work, for example), emotional tensions, colds and other respiratory infections, various foods (chocolate, nuts, seafood), and, in rare instances, menstruation.

If left alone, the blisters rupture and form small ulcerations. The ulcers then form crusts and scabs and finally heal in 10 to 14 days. As a rule, they do not leave scars.

If there is excessive pain or discomfort and the lymph glands in the neck become swollen, it usually means the virus has caused a secondary infection. When this happens, an oral antibiotic may be necessary.

We know of no single, effective cure for cold sores and fever blisters. Many o-t-c remedies, however, are often effective in relieving the signs and symptoms of cold sores of the mouth and lips. A new product—Resolve (Dow)—is the latest topical medication that affords relief from this annoying disorder.

If your cold sores are persistent or recurring, it is wise to consult your physician. In extreme cases, herpes simplex has been known to cause complications and produce disease in the eyes, brain, and internal organs.

Genital Herpes

Since cold sores of the genital area are transmitted by sexual contact, this condition is considered a venereal disease. Attacking over 500,000 Americans each year, genital herpes is reportedly the most prevalent venereal disease among young Americans today, its incidence being greater than both gonorrhea and syphilis.

Like cold sores about the mouth and lips, genital herpes is transmitted by a virus. Given the opportunity, this virus can infect—by direct contact—any portion of the body surface of a susceptible individual. What is particularly disturbing are the unpredictable recurrences of these genital infections in the same person—at the same site—with a frequency that can be distressing, embarrassing and, at times, disabling.

How do you know if you have genital herpes? The average incubation period—that is, from the time of contact to symptoms — is roughly a week. At this time, any number of signs and symptoms may precede or accompany a herpes infection of the genital region. These can include itching, mild burning and prickling sensations, pain during urination and intercourse, fever, headache, and swollen lymph glands in the groin area.

Small blisters, in groups, commonly appear at the infected site—usually around the vagina or on the penis. These break down in a few days leaving painful, shallow ulcers which, when not complicated by any other infection, heal in about a week or ten days.

A genital herpes infection can be a painful, swollen, inflammatory process in some and a relatively mild, transient, and asymptomatic one in others. Those who are completely asymptomatic—and there are many—may act as reservoirs, or "carriers," for the disease, unknowingly affecting any and all sex partners.

And so the question often posed by a spouse, "Who gave you (me) this herpes infection?", cannot be answered. (I call this a marital argument that starts from scratch!)

Someone developing a herpetic infection a week after sex relations has not necessarily contracted herpes from his or her sex partner. The friction of intercourse may very well have activated a dormant herpes virus in his or her body.

And while the primary infection (meaning the first time one is afflicted with the condition) is acquired by direct sexual contact, (genital to genital or mouth to genital), recurrences of genital herpes infections generally represent reactivation of a latent, hidden virus, rather than reinfection.

What causes these reactivations—these recurrences—and what are some of the triggering mechanisms? No one really knows.

After an active herpes episode, the virus retreats to and remains quietly hidden in a nerve root, thus making treatment difficult if not impossible. After a period of weeks, months, or even years, the virus, stirred up by any number of mechanisms, travels down the nerve path and reappears on the skin, starting up a new batch of small blisters with all the accompanying symptoms of the earlier herpes infection. Some of the reactivating mechanisms that have been implicated in provoking recurrences include mechanical trauma, masturbation, sexual intercourse, fever, gastrointestinal upsets, sunburn, fatigue, overexertion, sleeplessness, poor nutrition, menstruation, psychic stress, and even sauna baths!

What is most disturbing about genital herpes is its serious consequences.

Extensive herpes of the genital organs can cause excruciating pain during urination and sexual intercourse.

During pregnancy, where genital herpes is three times more frequent than in non-pregnant women, it results in a higher incidence of miscarriage and a greater likelihood of prematurity. If active genital herpes is present at the time of delivery, it can cause a devastating or fatal infection in the newborn as the infant passes through the birth canal.

In addition, women with herpesvirus Type 2 infections run a five times greater risk of cancer of the cervix than those without genital herpes.

And for both women and men who have genital herpes, the incidence of other venereal infections is much higher than for those in the general population.

While effective treatment for herpes is poor at best, you should consult your physician to try to prevent complications that could lead to severe secondary bacterial infection and wide dissemination of the disease.

Treatment of the active infection consists mainly of supportive therapy:

- Relieve the inflammation and swelling with tepid baths or continuous compresses using cool, whole milk.
- Eliminate the subjective symptoms of pain and itching with aspirin and antihistamines and appropriate local medications prescribed by your physician.
- Control any secondary bacterial and yeast infections—again with medications prescribed by your doctor.
- Since urine will cause unmerciful pain and stinging of vulvar lesions in women, protect those delicate areas with zinc oxide paste.

As far as specific treatments, there are as many different kinds as there are physicians. Everything works...and nothing works...

Past and present therapies have included idoxuridine, commonly called IDU, in the form of an ointment; various cortisone-like antibiotic creams and ointments; and applications of ice cubes, liquid nitrogen, ether, chloroform, nail polish remover, ethyl chloride in the form of a spray, cortisone-type sprays, and a dozen different other topical preparations.

Some doctors recommend photodynamic inactivation, or the so-called "dye-light" therapy, where the external lesions are painted with a dye that has the ability to make the virus sensitive to light. After painting on the solution (dye), the lesions are exposed to ordinary light which purportedly inactivates the virus, thus shortening the clinical course of the disease.

Controlled studies, however, have found all these therapeutic measures wanting; some may even have undesirable side effects. For example, the safety of the technically simple and inexpensive photodye therapy, which has enjoyed quick and widespread popularity among physicians, is open to serious question at the present time.

The latest theory—still unproven, of course—suggests that a harmless amino acid, lysine, when taken orally for a period of six months, will prevent recurrences of herpes lesions. I have been recommending it to my patients in the form of Enisyl (3 tablets daily), and some of the results have been most encouraging.

Just as there are dozens of therapies for active lesions, so are there dozens of theories and modalities said to prevent recurrences. These include vaccine therapy with various vaccines, including smallpox, oral polio, and herpes vaccine. A new vaccine, Lupidon, is being used successfully in Europe and is said to prevent recurrences in 90 to 95% of the cases. Treatment consists of a total of 30 injections administered weekly for seven months and then monthly until the symptoms disappear. It has not been cleared by the Food and Drug Administration yet. Any physician in this country who administers Lupidon to patients who have brought it into the U.S. is subject to license revocation. It's a felony!

Another theory is that oral contraceptives help to prevent recurrences. Women taking the birth control pills are said to have fewer recurrences than women who do not. It is also said that the chemicals in most contraceptive foams, when used inside the vagina, have an anti-viral effect on the genital type of herpes virus.

Another recent study reports that a relatively non-toxic substance—deoxy-D-glucose—has been shown to be the latest, effective chemotherapeutic agent in the treatment of genital herpes.

Again, none of the above has yet withstood the test of time, but many physicians still swear by their particular system or technique.

Unfortunately, we cannot eradicate the virus by simply treating the local infection.

For those with genital herpes we are left with this sobering thought: those who have it, have it for life. And every time it recurs, it can potentially infect other people.

What, then, can be done to prevent dissemination of the disease to non-infected sex partners? Here are a few recommendations and suggestions:

- Practice good genital hygiene. That means "soap and water."
- Wear loose, soft clothing and avoid rubbing and chafing.
- For recurrence in uncircumsized men, circumcision is advised.
- When oral or genital lesions are present, don't have sex.

The cure for these herpes infections will ultimately come from an anti-viral antibiotic that will destroy the virus in its hidden, dormant lair—the nerve root. And if a safe vaccine could be produced—such as those given to children in a single dose—then herpes, like diphtheria, typhoid, polio, smallpox and influenza, could forever be eradicated.

We're working on it...

Treating Cold Sores

Home Remedies

Before the cold sore blisters appear, there may be a tingling and itchy sensation of the part that is affected. (For those with recurrent herpes infections, these are familiar signs.) To help reduce the size of the cold sore that will inevitably follow, try applying an ice cube to the area for about five minutes every half hour or so.

Applying acetone (nail polish remover), taking care not to inhale the fumes, will also give relief and/or shorten the duration of the infection.

Local Medications

There are also many over-the-counter cold sore preparations that may help if applied early. Try any of the following:

Resolve (Dow)
Campho-Phenique Liquid or **Gel** (Winthrop)
Blistex Ointment (Blistex)
Cold Sore Lotion (De Witt)

You can also ask your friendly pharmacist to give you a bottle of the following:

Camphor Spirit (N.F.)

Directions: Apply with Q-Tips every 3 or 4 hours.

Sunscreens

If your cold sores are precipitated by exposure to the sun, use a sunscreen or sunblock in the form of a cream, lotion or gel before you go out into the sun. (See chapter on Sun-Poisoning, page 123.) I also recommend using one of the following sun-screening "lipsticks":

PreSun Sunscreen Lip Protection (Westwood)
Sun Stick (Cooper)

RVPaba Lipstick (Elder)
Eclipse Sunscreen Lip & Face Protectant (Herbert)

Oral Medications

For some people, taking two aspirins a couple of hours before exposure to the sun often will prevent sun-induced herpes of the lips. In addition, the following oral medication has shown encouraging results in preventing recurrences of cold sores.

Enisyl 500 mg (Person and Covey)

Directions: 3 tablets daily for a period of 6 months may prevent recurrences of herpes lesions.

Shingles

Shingles is an inflammation of a nerve which causes pain, itching, a rash, or all three.

It has nothing to do with "nerves" in the emotional sense. People are often heard to say, "Oh! She's very nervous so she came down with the shingles." Poppycock. Because shingles affects a *nerve,* many people mistake this to mean that it is a nervous condition.

The condition has afflicted its share of celebrities—Golda Meir immediately comes to mind—and that notoriety also has led to many misconceptions about it.

Shingles, the technical name for which is herpes zoster, is caused by a virus. It's the same virus that is responsible for chicken pox. Unlike chicken pox, however, it is only slightly contagious.

Although shingles can affect any age group, it's more prevalent and more painful in older people. Depending upon the severity and the location of the nerve involved, shingles can be mistaken in its early stages for attacks of appendicitis, kidney stones, gallbladder trouble, pleurisy, and even facial neuralgia and toothache.

The virus of shingles attacks a nerve root in the brain or spinal cord and follows the course of that nerve only. Early symptoms include a feeling of fatigue, headache, a slight fever, and a mild drawing pain over the involved area. They may be followed by itching and a rash of small blisters, usually in groups, along the affected nerve.

Since each nerve extends to a very specific part of the body, the blisters usually have a ribbon-like or branching configuration forming a semi-circle on one side of the body.

Since shingles can attack any peripheral nerve, it may localize on the scalp, face, trunk, or an extremity. Shingles occurring along a nerve at the lower part of the back of the neck will affect an arm, forearm and hand. If it attacks a nerve in the middle of the back, the symptoms will spread around one side of the body to the belly-button or thereabouts. If it disturbs the nerves at the lower end of the spinal column (the sacral area), it will affect the entire lower extremity on that side. No area of the body surface is immune.

In children, shingles usually runs a mild and quick course, and the average victim will recover without any type of therapy. In older persons, however, the pain may become excruciating, the itching may be intense, and the blisters may become crusted and infected.

Since there can be complications arising from even the mildest form of shingles, it is important that a physician examine any suspected case.

Your doctor can prescribe various internal medications, such as antibiotics, cortisone-like drugs, analgesics, and antihistamines, to relieve the pain, itching, and inflammation and soothing salves and ointments to relieve the dermatitis and possibly prevent spread of the disease. When shingles involves the eye, you should consult an ophthalmologist (a physician who specializes in diseases of the eye) to prevent irreparable damage to the cornea.

Other complications of shingles which may occur are scarring where the blisters were, persistent dull or severe pain (post-herpetic neuralgia) which may linger for months or longer after the rash has disappeared, and extreme fatigue and malaise during the period of recovery.

At the present time there are no measures known to prevent shingles. You may save yourself some worry, however, by avoiding direct contact with someone who has shingles. If you are older, and therefore more susceptible to shingles, you should also avoid young children who have chicken pox. Doctors will sometimes prescribe gamma globulin for patients who are otherwise very ill and who have been exposed to persons who have either chicken pox or shingles.

Shingles almost always limits itself to one side of the body. So, if you have a rash on both sides, chances are that shingles is not the culprit.

Treating Shingles

Compresses

For the early, blistery eruption, use soothing compresses or wet dressings to help relieve the inflammation, allay the itching and dry up the blisters. Follow the directions for applying wet dressings on page 208, using any of the following:

AluWets Wet Dressing Crystals (Stiefel)
Directions: Dissolve contents of one packet in 12 ounces of warm water and apply as open wet dressings for 15 to 20 minutes every 2 to 3 hours.

Bluboro Powder (Herbert)
Directions: Dissolve contents of one packet in 1 pint (16 ounces) of warm water and apply as above.

Domeboro Powder (Dome)
Directions: Dissolve contents of one packet in 1 pint (16 ounces) of warm water and apply as above.

Dalidome Powder Packets (Dome)
Directions: Dissolve contents of one packet in 1 pint (16 ounces) of warm water and apply as above.

Anti-Itch Medications

Following the compresses, and when the blisters are still present, you may want to apply a soothing, cooling lotion to help reduce the inflammation and stop the itching. Ask your pharmacist to make up the following:

Phenol **½%**
Calamine Lotion (USP) **to make 8 oz.**
Directions: Apply this every 3 to 4 hours using your fingers or a soft, one-inch, flat varnish paint brush.

The compresses aren't necessary once the blisters have begun to dry up. At this point, apply a less drying form of medication. Ask your pharmacist to make up the following:

Phenol	**½%**
Calamine Liniment (USP)	**to make 8 oz.**

Directions: Apply this every 3 to 4 hours.

When the lesions have all dried up, but the itching remains, try an anti-itch preparation such as the following and apply it whenever necessary for itching:

Rhulicort Cream (Lederle)

Or, ask your druggist to grind up and mix the following for you:

Menthol	**¼%**
Phenol	**½%**
Cold Cream	**to make 2 oz.**

Directions: Apply this preparation every 3 or 4 hours for the itching.

Oral Medications

If the itching persists despite the local measures described above, an antihistamine preparation will often provide relief. One of the very few non-prescription antihistamines is:

Chlor-Trimeton Tablets 4 mg (Schering)

Directions: Take one tablet every 4 hours to relieve mild to moderate itching. (Chlor-Trimeton also comes in syrup form and can be purchased in 4-ounce bottles. One teaspoonful contains 2 mg of the antihistamine, which is one-half the tablet dose.)

For accompanying pain, use any analgesic (aspirin, Bufferin, Anacin, Excedrin, etc.), in appropriate dosage.

Note Well: If your shingles:

- Occurs in the area about the eye
- Is extensive
- Appears infected
- Is extremely painful or itchy, or
- Is unresponsive to the therapy outlined above

see your physician at once.

Impetigo

Impetigo is a highly contagious, unsightly skin infection caused by the staphylococcus and streptococcus bacteria. The medical term for this condition, appropriately, is impetigo contagiosa.

Impetigo can be recognized by a thick, stuck-on, honey-colored crust which usually appears around the nostrils and mouth, although any portion of the skin surface may be affected. It occurs primarily in children, but adults can fall victim, too, usually by direct contact with infected children.

Impetigo begins on damaged skin, when the outer protective layers are damaged and the normal resistance of the skin lowered by cuts, bruises, insect bites, or other skin diseases, such as chicken pox, cold sores, or acne. Healthy skin seems to act as a barrier to suppress these harmful bacteria.

The mouth and nose, which suffer constant rubbing and wiping, are the prime areas on which impetigo begins. The infectious germs are carried to other parts of the body by dirty fingers and fingernails and by unclean towels, utensils, and clothing. They can also spread to other people who have direct contact with infected persons, especially through kissing, wrestling, or other such contact sports.

Once impetigo takes hold, it spreads very easily—even to normal healthy skin—and may last for several weeks. If not controlled, it can lead to internal infections accompanied by fever, fatigue, and swollen lymph glands.

Those infected with impetigo should seek prompt medical attention. A doctor's care can help prevent generalized spread, especially to other members of the family and friends, and possibly prevent the serious internal complications that may arise, such as kidney infections.

Treatment consists of gently removing the crusts and thoroughly cleansing the affected areas 4 times daily with an appropriate *antibacterial* soap. One good antibacterial soap is pHisoHex, which can be obtained only with a prescription from your physician. There also are some over-the-counter soaps with antiseptic properties that may be effective. If the crusts stick stubbornly to the underlying skin, you may need to apply warm water compresses to lift them off.

After each thorough washing, rub an antibiotic ointment into the affected area. *Do not cover the area with bandages or gauze.* Exposure to air will help kill many types of germs and speed the healing process.

If the condition is extensive and severe, your physician may prescribe an oral antibiotic, such as penicillin or erythromycin, or a penicillin injection.

The following are some additional measures that help eliminate impetigo and prevent its spread:

- Wash hands thoroughly and frequently with antibacterial soap.
- Keep fingernails trimmed and scrupulously clean at all times.
- Change towels and bed linen daily.
- Isolate infected person from other individuals until all the crusts have disappeared (usually 2 or 3 days). This includes keeping children home during the acute, crusted stage of the disease.
- Wash the infected person's laundry separately, and make sure no one else uses his or her soap, towels, or linens.
- Continue treatment for 7 to 10 days after all the crusts are gone.

If after several days of therapy the lesions persist, contact your physician regarding further treatment.

Treating Impetigo

In the superficial variety of impetigo, seen on the face and caused mainly by the staphylococcal organisms, many physicians believe that thorough cleansing and good, topical therapy—without oral or injectable antibiotics—can do the trick.

Soaps & Cleansers

Wash the affected areas thoroughly three or four times daily with one of the following antibacterial soaps:

Dial (Armour)
Safeguard (Procter & Gamble)

Or use this antiseptic cleanser:

Hibiclens (Stuart)

Local Medications

After thorough washing, gently remove any crusts that are *loosely* attached (this is best done with a clean, washed tweezers). Then apply one of the following antibacterial preparations at least 3 times daily:

Mycitracin Ointment (Upjohn)
Neosporin Ointment (Burroughs Wellcome)

Continue the washing and ointment applications for at least a week after the crusts have disappeared.

If the lesions persist despite the adequate treatment outlined above, see your physician at once.

Note: Some physicians recommend the administration of oral or injectable antibiotics for the treatment of impetigo to prevent some of the rare complications, such as kidney infections.

Athlete's Foot

Athlete's foot does attack the feet. But it by no means is limited to athletes. It is also known as ringworm. But it is not a worm.

Having disposed of two popular misconceptions about this ailment that gets a toe-hold on so many people, let's get down to what it really is.

Athlete's foot is a nasty infection caused by a fungus. It occurs mostly among adult males. It is fairly easy to treat—but it can be stubborn, too.

Fungous infections, or diseases caused by a fungus, are among the most common skin disorders in the world. Fungi are living germs—actually miniature plants—which grow and multiply on the skin, in the hair, and on the nails of most all living creatures.

Why certain people develop fungous infections and others do not are questions that have not yet been resolved. There is speculation that some individuals are immune to certain types of infections, and ringworm may be one of these.

The reason for its lower incidence in females is unknown. Perhaps women are cleaner, sweat less, wash more often, and wear looser footgear. Maybe their hormones have anti-fungal properties. We really don't know.

Ringworm of the feet does not occur in primitive races accustomed to going barefoot, and it almost never appears in children under the age of 12. Thus, if your child has a rash on his or her feet, it probably is *not* a fungous infection.

The fungus of athlete's foot may be present on the skin of the feet without causing any infection or other symptoms. It is only when the natural resistance of the skin is lowered that the fungi thrive, proliferate, invade the outer layers of the skin, and set up housekeeping. This lowered resistance may be the result of excessive moisture and sweating (particularly in the summertime, due to sweaty socks and not drying your feet after swimming and bathing), inadequate ventilation of the feet (tight shoes and socks), uncleanliness, or friction.

Athlete's foot affects people in different ways. For some it is characterized by peeling, cracking, and scaling of the toe webs (particularly the last toe web). Others experience redness, scaling, and blisters along the sides and soles of their feet. Occasionally there is intense itching. By the way, every eruption on the feet is not necessarily athlete's foot. It may be a contact allergy (from shoes and dyes), psoriasis, or any of a number of conditions that frequently attack the feet and toes.

If you have a persistent rash on your feet, consult your physician. Over-the-counter medications may only aggravate conditions that have been misdiagnosed as athlete's foot. And, if left untreated, athlete's foot can lead to infection by other organisms (bacteria), which may require antibiotic therapy, continuous wet dressings, and complete bed rest. Only your doctor can diagnose athlete's foot with any certainty.

Once diagnosed, treatment should be instituted without delay. In the simple, uncomplicated cases, this involves applying anti-fungal creams twice daily. The creams should relieve the symptoms fairly rapidly and usually cure the condition in a matter of weeks. In acute cases, where there is weeping, oozing, and blister formation and the toe webs are wet and soggy, you should soak your feet twice a day in potassium permanganate solution (a prescription item) before applying the anti-fungal cream.

If your athlete's foot is stubborn, persistent, and extensive, or if you have an allergic spread on your fingers and hands in the form of itchy water blisters, your physician will usually prescribe anti-fungal medication to be taken by mouth.

In addition to the local and oral medicines, these rules are important:

- Wash your feet at least once daily.
- Keep them meticulously dry at all times.
- Wear only cotton socks.
- Avoid tight or snug footwear in hot, humid weather (perforated shoes or sandals are preferable).
- Dust an anti-fungal powder into your shoes in the summertime.

If you follow these directions, you will never be tripped up by athlete's foot.

Treating Athlete's Foot

Soaking

In the acute stage, when your toe webs and toes are red, oozing and blistered, do not apply creams or ointments. The only helpful therapy is to soak in antiseptic solutions every 4 to 6 hours. See page 209 for the proper method to soak feet and hands. Use any of the following:

AluWets Wet Dressing Crystals (Stiefel)
Bluboro Powder (Herbert)
Domeboro Powder Packets (Dome)

During the soaking process, keep your toe webs separated by thin strips of linen or cotton material, such as old, washed sheeting or shirting. Never use cotton balls or batting, as their wood fiber content can be irritating.

Creams

During the subacute stage, when the lesions have begun to dry up, apply either of the following to the affected areas twice daily:

Tinactin Cream (Schering)
Vioform Cream 3% (Ciba)

Note: This last preparation stains somewhat and is not as effective as the Tinactin Cream.

Powder

Dust the following powder on your feet twice daily:

Zeasorb Powder (Stiefel)

It is important to keep the toes separated at this phase of treatment as well. Use lamb's wool, purchased from your pharmacist, day and night.

Ointments

For the chronic variety of athlete's foot, with thick scaling of the soles and sides of the feet, have your pharmacist make up the following:

Whitfield's Ointment (one-half strength)

Directions: Apply to affected areas twice daily.

Insect Bites and Stings

Spring and summer mean lush foliage, sunshine, flowers and...The Sting.

For those who work or play in the fields and gardens, bees, wasps, hornets, and yellow jackets buzz around loaded with nuisance, pain, and sometimes danger.

Bites and stings, for the most part, are only an annoyance and rarely cause more than slight, temporary discomfort. However, toxic or allergic reactions to insect stings occasionally can be fatal in sensitive individuals. In fact, there are more deaths in the United States from insect stings than from snake bites.

The reactions of insect stings are due either to allergic mechanisms or to the release of certain chemicals, toxins, or enzymes in the venom.

The honeybee and yellow jacket are responsible for most stings. Although they may have similar appearances, these two insects have very different habits. The honeybee is a social insect that uses a stinger to inject venom into its victim. A yellow jacket is a wasp which can both bite and sting. The honeybee presents a special problem as the only insect that leaves its stinger and venom sac in the victim.

The average, simple, normal sting, the one most commonly encountered, is accompanied by varying degrees of localized pain lasting for a few minutes. This is followed by redness, swelling (in the form of a wheal or hive), and itching of the affected part. If no complications arise, all traces of the sting will usually disappear within a few hours.

In the exaggerated type of local reaction, there is more itching as well as increased swelling which causes some distortion of the area involved. Also, the condition may last longer, and there may be a great deal of discomfort.

The treatment for most insect bites and stings is the same. However, in the case of a bee sting, it is vitally important to remove the barbed stinger and attached venom sac as quickly as possible, as contractions of the walls of the sac continue to inject venom for a period of time.

Never try pulling the stinger out or squeezing the area in which the stinger has been embedded. This will break the venom sac, releasing more of the toxic or allergic substances and markedly aggravating the symptoms. Rather, gently scrape with a knife blade or fingernail until the stinger and sac have been dislodged.

After you remove the stinger and venom sac, follow these steps for the simple insect sting:

- Wash the affected area with soap and water.
- Use ice packs or cold compresses for 30 to 45 minutes to reduce the inflammation and swelling.
- Apply a paste made up of equal parts of unseasoned meat tenderizer and water to the affected area (wheal). This often results in prompt, lasting relief.
- Treat any hives and itching by applying phenolated calamine lotion every 3 or 4 hours.
- If severe swelling, itching, and pain persist, call your physician. You may need an antihistamine or cortisone-like drug to counteract the bee venom.
- If you're stung on your foot or leg, elevate it and keep it at rest.

How Best To Avoid Insect Bites and Stings

- Always wear shoes outside. Bare feet are the most vulnerable areas for insect attacks. (Bees love clover and yellow jackets live in the ground.)

- Avoid scented soaps, perfumes, colognes, and other toiletries as these odors attract insects.
- Wear light-colored, smooth fabrics; avoid bright, flowery prints and dark, rough clothing. These, too, attract insects.
- Avoid bright jewelry and other metal objects.
- Avoid touching insect nests.
- Keep house screens in good repair.
- Keep garbage cans covered at all times.
- Use insect repellants on exposed parts of your body and on your clothing.

Treating Bites

Home Remedies

For a few, localized insect bites, where there is redness, swelling, and itching, the best immediate treatment is applying ice. An ice cube, held on the bite areas for 5 or 10 minutes, will usually give prompt relief of the pain, itching, and swelling.

Another good "home remedy" is the application of a paste made up of equal parts of unseasoned meat tenderizer and water. A half-teaspoonful of each, applied to the bite, can quickly relieve the symptoms.

Local Medications

The following is another preparation that may be used for the localized variety of insect bites:

Rhulicort Cream (Lederle)

Directions: Apply every 3 or 4 hours to the affected areas.

You also can ask your pharmacist to make up the following:

Menthol	**¼%**
Phenol	**1%**
Cold Cream	**to make 2 oz.**

Directions: Apply every 2 to 3 hours to the bites.

Baths

For multiple or widespread insect bites, soothing baths usually work best. Any of the following should give relief:

Aveeno Oilated (Cooper)
Alpha Keri Therapeutic Bath Oil (Westwood)
nutraSpa (Owen)

Directions: Follow the directions on the labels.

Lotions

The baths may be followed by the following preparation:

Rhulicort Lotion (Lederle)

Directions: Apply every 3 or 4 hours for itching.

Or have your pharmacist compound the following:

Phenol ½%
Calamine Lotion **to make 8 oz.**

Directions: Apply every 3 or 4 hours for itching.

Or, try:

Campho-Phenique Liquid (Winthrop)

Directions: Same as above.

Oral Medications

To relieve the itching of insect bites and stings, use the following over-the-counter antihistamine. It may cause drowsiness, so read the label for dosage and warnings.

Chlor-Trimeton Tablets 4 mg (Schering)

If none of these remedies relieves your symptoms, consult your physician.

Hives

Hives is a very common disorder. At least 20 percent of the general population will develop some form of hive-like eruption in the course of a lifetime.

What is hives? Contrary to popular opinion, it is *not* a disease. Caused by the release of a chemical called histamine, hives, or what is known medically as urticaria, is a symptom of some disorder or allergic mechanism going on in the body. Hives appears on the skin and mucous membranes in the form of itching, stinging, and burning wheals (or welts), surrounded by a zone of redness. It comes in a variety of sizes, shapes, and locations.

When the wheals are very large—and when portions of the eyelids and lips swell up to cause actual disfigurement—the condition is called angioneurotic edema, or "bull hives." Hives also may involve the mucous membranes of the mouth and throat, and in rare cases may even obstruct breathing so severely that heroic medical measures are required to prevent suffocation.

Like coughing or sneezing, which may signal a response to an upper respiratory infection, hay-fever, and the like, hives is a clue which alerts us to abnormal goings-on in our system. For example, it may be a response to an infection, an allergic reaction to some strange food or drug, or emotional tension.

Hives is one of the most difficult conditions for which to find a specific cause, mainly because the possibilities are endless. In the acute type of hives—where the itching and wheals appear quickly and fade in a few minutes or hours—it is somewhat easier to uncover the precise cause: a strange food, an emotional upset, a penicillin injection, a new medication. Unfortunately, this isn't the case in trying to determine the cause for the chronic form. This chronic form occurs most commonly in middle-aged women and may last for months or years.

The most common causes of hives are related to foods and drugs. Strawberries, nuts, fish and shellfish, milk, eggs, pork, oranges, bananas, and many other edibles can cause hives.

Of the various drugs and medications, penicillin is probably the most common cause. People who are allergic to penicillin and suffer from hives should avoid milk and certain cheeses (such as bleu cheese and Roquefort). Milk and other dairy products may contain sufficient penicillin to keep hives alive for years. Not only is this drug given to sick cattle for infections, but it is frequently dumped into the large milk vats in an attempt to lower the bacterial counts in order to conform to certain health standards. Caveat emptor!

Another common cause is aspirin. When you realize that about 15 million pounds of aspirin are consumed in the United States each year, it's little wonder that we see so many reactions from it.

Related to aspirin are other hive-producing chemicals known as salicylates. Salicylates can be found in such products as root beer, wintergreen and mint flavorings, commercial bakery products, and mixes. Certain food dyes and preservatives (such as sodium benzoate), insulin, and various vaccines to protect against measles and polio may also be common offenders. So is menthol, found in such diverse products as cigarettes, toothpaste, candies, jellies, Noxzema, room deodorants, lozenges, and shaving creams.

Some people get hives from inhaling substances such as animal dander (from cats, dogs or horses), house dust, pollen, molds, certain plants, and flour in bakeries. Others break out in hives when they touch something cold or when they touch something hot and still others when they are exposed to sunlight. Some even get hives when pressure is applied to their skin, as in the shower.

There are certain types of hives which are known to be of psychogenic origin. Fear, anger, and stress are the primary psychological factors responsible.

The treatment of hives consists of identifying and eliminating the cause of the condition. You—the patient—must be the detective. What food did you eat? What medication did you take? Where were you just before the wheals appeared? Anything new? Anything different? Have you been in some strange place? What different inhalants or sprays have you been exposed to lately?

See your doctor if your hives are persistent, recurring, or severe. It is important that you ask yourself all these questions mentioned above and provide as much information as you can to your physician. Only a physician can unearth the origin and nature of your hives, and only a physician can eradicate them. You may need a thorough physical examination, blood tests, X-rays, allergy testing, and other laboratory examinations to rule out any internal infection, such as hepatitis.

For acute, temporary hives, prescription antihistamines (such as Tacaryl or Atarax), given by mouth, usually relieve the symptoms promptly—at least until your next exposure to the culprit. Chronic, recurrent cases require patience, extensive detective work, and often hospitalization to hunt down the precise source of the urticarial eruption.

Only when the cause has been revealed can hives be controlled.

Treating Hives

Until you've identified and eliminated the culprit that's causing your hives, you can try to ease its annoying symptoms.

Baths

To soothe and decrease the itching of generalized hives, take lukewarm baths in any of the following bath preparations:

Alpha Keri Therapeutic Bath Oil (Westwood)
Aveeno Oilated Bath (Cooper)
nutraSpa Bath Oil (Owen)
Directions: Follow directions on the labels.

Creams & Lotions

Following the bath, apply the following preparation every 3 or 4 hours:

Rhulicort Cream (Lederle)

Or ask your pharmacist to make up one of the following:

Phenol **½%**
Calamine Lotion (USP) **to make 4 oz.**
Directions: Apply every 3 to 4 hours using your fingers or a soft, one-inch, flat varnish paint brush.

Menthol **¼%**
Phenol **½%**
Cold Cream **to make 2 oz.**
Directions: Apply this soothing and cooling preparation every 3 or 4 hours for itching.

Oral Medications

If you need extra relief from itching, try the following antihistamine:

Chlor-Trimeton Tablets 4 mg (Schering)
Directions: Take one tablet every 3 or 4 hours. Check the cautions on the label.

Pityriasis Rosea

Pityriasis rosea is one of the most perplexing skin disorders. No one knows what causes it or what makes it disappear in a matter of weeks. But we do know that it isn't contagious.

Pityriasis rosea has no common name. It comes from the Greek and Latin words for "fine, pink scaling," which appropriately describe its appearance. Although commonly mistaken for ringworm, pityriasis rosea is unique. It usually begins as a single, large, round or oval pinkish patch, known as the "mother" or "herald" plaque. This patch is followed in 10 to 14 days by a blossoming of small, flat, oval, scaly patches of similar hue, usually distributed in a Christmas tree pattern over the chest and back.

This fairly generalized eruption seldom itches and usually limits itself to areas from the neck to the knees. It occurs more frequently in adolescents and young adults and in the spring and autumn. It disappears as mysteriously as it came in about 6 to 8 weeks, without leaving any scars or marks and without causing any complications. It almost never recurs. It rarely crops up in the same family at the same time, it is not a sign of ill health, and it doesn't affect the unborn children of pregnant women who are afflicted with it.

In other words, it's a pretty friendly skin condition!

There are, of course, exceptions to all the above facts, as there are in most skin diseases. For example, the herald plaque, which is supposed to signal the coming of a batch of smaller lesions, may be neither large nor evident. Also, while the normal rash, at its peak, consists of individual lesions in a patterned distribution, it may cover the entire body. Occasionally, the condition may be accompanied by fierce and uncontrollable itching, and, even more rarely, by fever, malaise, loss of appetite, and swollen lymph glands in the neck.

I have seen pityriasis rosea last for over three months, and I've seen cases in the summer and winter. Several of my patients have been young children in whom not only the trunk but the entire face and scalp were covered with fine, intensely itchy bumps, and I've even noted recurrences of this condition time and again.

But, fortunately these are only the exceptions. Usually, it is a relatively mild condition.

The treatment of pityriasis rosea is purely symptomatic. If it doesn't itch, leave it alone. If your itching is only slight, soothing baths and plain calamine lotion applied 2 or 3 times daily should give you adequate relief. However, if the itching becomes intense and the rash begins to spread very rapidly, you should consult your physician, who will prescribe appropriate oral medication and sometimes ultraviolet light treatments to relieve the itching and possibly shorten the course of the disease.

One last bit of advice: For your own peace of mind, don't take too much stock in non-professional diagnosis. Some patients, noting the sudden onset and generalized spread of this strange rash, have shown it to relatives, friends, and the friendly pharmacist, only to be told that they probably have either ringworm, syphilis, or some bizarre blood disorder. The most important consideration for those with pityriasis rosea is the reassurance that it is neither serious, contagious, infectious, nor malignant and it will eventually disappear in a matter of a few weeks without leaving permanent marks or scars.

Treating Pityriasis Rosea

Baths

Since pityriasis rosea is usually fairly widespread, the best method of treating it is with soothing baths. For the scaling and the itching that accompany it, use any of the following:

Alpha Keri Therapeutic Bath Oil (Westwood)
Aveeno Oilated Bath (Cooper)
nutraSpa Bath Oil (Owen)

Local Medications

If the itching persists, apply either of the following:

Schamberg's Lotion (C & M Pharmacal)
Rhulicort Lotion (Lederle)

Or have your pharmacist compound this:

Menthol	**¼%**
Phenol	**½%**
Mī-Skin Lotion	**to make 8 oz.**

Directions for all three: Apply to the affected areas 2 or 3 times daily.

If there are only a few itchy spots, apply the following:

Rhulicort Cream (Lederle)

Directions: Apply to the affected areas 2 or 3 times daily.

For any dryness that remains after the condition runs its course, use one of the following 2 or 3 times daily:

Keri Lotion (Westwood)
Carmol-10 Lotion (Syntex)
LactiCare Lotion (Stiefel)
Nutraplus Lotion (Owen)

Oral Medications

If these measures don't relieve the itching, take this antihistamine every 4 hours as necessary:

Chlor-Trimeton Tablets 4 mg (Schering)

Infestations

While parasitic infestations of the human skin are not considered common afflictions in the United States, there are two types of organisms which have recently caused virtual epidemics. These organisms—called ectoparasites—are lice and mites.

Infestations with lice (true insects) and mites (insect-like organisms) cause intensely itchy, annoying skin problems. Unless diagnosed and treated properly, these conditions can persist and eventually spread to family members, classmates, and friends.

Lice

Lice are small, wingless insects measuring about one-eighth of an inch in length. They have been around for centuries and have flourished without respect for social class or position.

Associated with wars and disease in the Middle Ages, lice carry typhus, a disease which has been known to wipe out entire armies. They were extremely prevalent throughout the world until World War II, at which time DDT almost eradicated this annoying and dread pestilence. However, the recent ban on DDT as a hazardous substance, along with the increase in social contact and world travel, have contributed to a resurgence of louse infestation throughout the world.

Today lice have become a major public health problem. Aggravated by poor living conditions, lack of personal cleanliness, and overcrowding, this infestation has reached epidemic proportions in many communities throughout the nation.

The main symptom of louse infestation—known technically as pediculosis—is a relentless "maddening itch" which is due to the salivary excretions of the culpable louse.

There are three kinds of lice affecting three different body areas: head lice, body lice, and pubic lice (also known as "crab" lice). Although each type has a different shape, they all feed by biting the skin and sucking the blood. The head louse attaches itself to the scalp. The body louse lives only in clothing. The crab louse attacks the hairs of the pubic region as well as the eyelashes.

The adult female louse lays eggs (nits) which she attaches with a glue-like substance to hairs or fibers of clothing. The eggs hatch in about ten days and reach maturity in about two weeks. Lice have a life span of about a month.

Head lice have become especially prevalent in recent years, particularly among school children in heavily populated areas. They make their home in your hair, causing intense itching and scratching of the scalp, the back of the neck, and behind the ears. In severe cases the lymph glands in the neck may become swollen. For some reason, head lice are almost never seen in blacks.

Looking closely, one sees small, silvery egg cases firmly attached to an individual hair shaft. Usually these nits will be close to the scalp—no more than a half-inch from where the hair begins. Although they resemble the scales of dandruff, they are much more difficult to remove than dandruff flakes because of the sticky, cement-like substance the female louse secretes to attach the nits.

Head lice are transmitted by direct contact with an infested person, by personal items such as combs, brushes, and pillow cases, and through clothing such as hats, scarves, ribbons, and other head coverings. If one person in a family or classroom has head lice, there is a good possibility that others in the same home or class will have it too.

Once your physician has established the diagnosis of head lice, treatment is relatively simple and highly effective. A prescription shampoo containing gamma benzene hexachloride (Kwell Shampoo) will cure a case of head lice in five minutes. One shampoo for five minutes. That's it! There is, in addition, a non-prescription shampoo called Vonce which works about as well.

After shampooing, you still may see eggs attached to the hair shaft, but these are now dead. To get rid of the unsightly but harmless dead nits, apply dilute vinegar (one-half vinegar and one-half water) to the scalp hair to loosen them and then back comb with a fine-tooth comb.

To prevent the spread of lice, thoroughly wash all articles of clothing that are suspected of having nits or adult lice. Also, use the Kwell Shampoo to clean combs, brushes, and other personal items of the affected person.

Kwell Lotion and Shampoo are also effective in treating both body and pubic lice.

Scabies

Scabies, like lice, has begun to reach epidemic proportions in the United States. Anybody and everybody can contact the disease. Poverty, with its crowded living conditions and poor hygiene, tends to promote the occurrence of scabies. However, there has been a definite increase of the disease in clean and fastidious individuals, the so-called "scabies of the cultivated," prompted, no doubt, by our changing morality and extensive worldwide travel.

Scabies is caused by a mite—a tiny creature, mistakenly referred to as an insect—which measures about one seventy-fifth of an inch in length, so small that it is barely visible to the naked eye. These mites burrow into the skin and spread from one individual to the next through personal and sexual contact. A different form of scabies found in animals (chiefly dogs) may be passed on to humans and cause a similar condition.

Scabies is characterized by intense itching, which is due to an allergy to the female mite and the eggs and feces she deposits underneath the upper layers of the skin. This itching is more apparent at night, when the tiny organisms become more active, and may increase when the person is overheated or removes his or her clothing. In many cases the itching is so intense that it leads to nervousness and loss of sleep.

Scabies may become generalized, but as a rule infections above the neck are extremely rare. The most common locations (the places the scabies mite is fond of attacking) are the webs of the fingers, the inner surfaces of the wrists, and the regions of the elbows. Other familiar locations where the mites set up housekeeping are the front of the armpits, the buttocks, the nipples, and the penis.

Too often scabies goes undiagnosed or misdiagnosed. Various topical salves and lotions may alleviate the itching for a short period of time. However, the infestation persists and the mites thrive, sometimes causing secondary infection which will require antibiotic therapy.

Once the proper diagnosis has been established—and only a physician is capable of recognizing it—the cure is relatively simple. Eurax Lotion and Kwell Lotion (prescription medications) will cure almost all cases of scabies with only one or two applications. (Kwell Lotion should not be used more than twice and should not be used in children under the age of six. Your doctor can tell you what other compounds are safe for very young children.) In addition, all contaminated clothing and linens should be thoroughly washed or dry cleaned.

Since scabies spreads so easily, it is vitally important that every person in a household affected by scabies be treated whether or not symptoms are present. All sex partners must be treated too.

So, for any persistent, widespread itching that is more pronounced at night and that is unrelieved by the usual simple baths and lotions, see your physician. Fortunately, the nasty scabies mite succumbs to a swift and simple cure.

Treating Lice

The following is a good, over-the-counter treatment for head lice:

Vonce Shampoo (Unipharm)

Directions: Apply Vonce Shampoo liberally to the scalp until entirely wet. Work into a lather and allow to remain on the hair and scalp for ten minutes, but not any longer. Rinse thoroughly with warm water and rub dry with a towel. Comb previously infested hairs thoroughly with a fine-tooth comb to remove dead lice and eggs (nits). Do not apply more than twice in any 24-hour period.

Treating Scabies

There are no over-the-counter remedies for scabies. If you suspect that you or members of your family have scabies or if you have had any recent contact with someone who had scabies, see your physician. He or she can make the diagnosis and prescribe the appropriate medication.

3 Contact Dermatitis

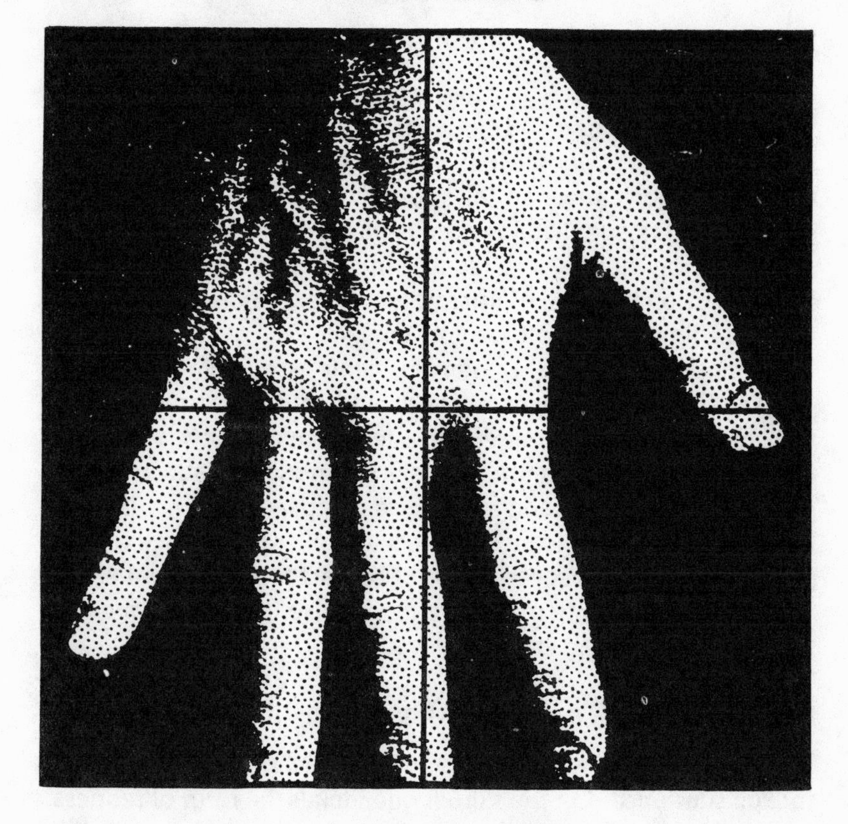

More and more, people of all ages and from all walks of life are exposed to thousands of different substances which can affect the skin through their use at home, work, or play. The tremendous increase in the number of new chemical-containing products found in industry and in the marketplace has been responsible for a large percentage of skin eruptions called contact dermatitis.

What do we mean by contact dermatitis? Simply stated, it is an inflammation of the skin which results from contact with any of a variety of natural or manufactured substances. The different types of contact dermatitis fall under two categories: reactions due to irritation and reactions due to allergy.

Reactions Due To Irritation (Primary Irritants)

A primary irritant is a substance strong enough to cause a demonstrable reaction and actual physical damage to the skin in a high percentage of people following initial exposure. It is similar in appearance to a mechanical injury or burn. Skin and deeper tissues are damaged, followed by inflammation and occasional scarring. How quickly the reaction occurs and how severe it is depends upon the type of irritant, its concentration, the length of exposure time, and the extent of contact.

Examples of strong primary irritants are lye, nitric acid, gasoline, turpentine, paint remover, and chemicals used for hair-straightening. These require only a few hours—or even minutes, in some cases—to injure the skin. And they affect almost everybody. Mild irritants, such as soaps, solvents, laundry bleaches, and metal cleansers, affect a smaller percentage of people and may require several days of contact to produce an effect.

Irritations due to chemicals are treated like burns. The aim is to soothe, comfort, and prevent infection and scarring.

Reactions Due To Allergy (Hypersensitivity)

In simple terms, an allergy is an overreaction of the body to a foreign substance. On the skin, it often takes the form of redness, itching, and swelling. In the respiratory system, it may take the form of hay-fever or asthma. In the intestinal tract, it may manifest itself as cramps and pains. And in the nervous system, it can result in migraine headaches.

The frequency of contact allergic skin rashes is not known, but it is estimated that of every 10 patients who see a physician for some skin problem, one will be diagnosed as having a contact dermatitis. Unlike the primary irritant dermatitis, allergic contact dermatitis requires a few days to a week before the symptoms appear.

The tendency to allergic skin reactions is unpredictable and varies from person to person. It may take repeated exposures to the same foreign substance for the skin cells to become sensitized and for a rash to appear. Some people can handle a substance for years without difficulty when suddenly, without notice or warning, they break out in a rash. Some people develop allergies to a large number of everyday products, while others never develop any signs of allergy. No one knows why.

There are myriad substances which all of us are exposed to in our daily lives that could conceivably cause an allergic dermatitis in otherwise healthy people. The majority of these substances can be found in the home or marketplace.

In wearing apparel:

- Wool, silk, furs, synthetic fibers, girdles, gloves, dress shields, stockings, and underwear elastic.
- Clothing additives and finishes applied to cloth to improve the look and feel—"wash and wear," permanent press, and anti-shrinkage and softening chemicals, especially the new fabric softeners used in clothes dryers, such as Bounce, Cling-Free, and Toss 'n Soft.
- Dyes—particularly the dark-brown, dark-blue, and black.
- Rubber materials, adhesives, chemicals used in the tanning of leather, and dyes in shoes. A dermatitis of the top of the feet and toes is almost invariably due to an allergy to something in the footwear, *not* athlete's foot.
- Leather goods, such as handbags, gloves, hatbands, and wallets.
- Parts of clothing and jewelry containing nickel, including rings, necklaces, earrings, bra clasps, garter clips, zippers, snaps, hairpins, and metal eyeglass frames.

Household items:

- Glues, paints and varnishes, waxes and polishes, oil stains, plastics, soaps, detergents, and household cleansers.
- Vegetables, fruit juices, and various spices.

In the garden:

- Plants—poison ivy, hyacinth, tulips, ragweed, etc.
- Chemicals—pesticides, insecticides, and fertilizers.

Over-the-counter drug preparations:

- Poison ivy remedies containing benzocaine and zirconium.
- Analgesic balms and liniments for burns, sunburn, and pain.
- Athlete's foot medications.
- Depilatory agents.
- Tar preparations for psoriasis and eczema.
- Anti-acne lotions, scrubs and salves, and a host of others.

Various parts of the body can be affected by certain materials more than others. For example, on the face, one should suspect cosmetics, nose drops, sprays, eyeglass frames, and over-the-counter salves and ointments. On the ears, consider earrings containing nickel (almost all do!), plastic hearing aids, hair dyes and sprays, perfumes, and other scented lotions. Allergic contact dermatitis of the neck can be caused by necklaces, hair dyes and sprays, collars, scarves, etc. In the armpits, consider antiperspirants, deodorants, and dress shields. For contact dermatitis of the lower extremities, think of socks, stockings, garters, pants, and shoes, as well as plants such as poison ivy. In the anal and genital areas, be aware of colored or perfumed toilet tissue, suppositories, hemorrhoid medications and various douches, deodorants, and contraceptive creams and devices. Hand eczemas are some of the most stubborn dermatoses known. Soaps, cleansers, detergents, gloves, plastics and a host of metals, plants, and chemicals may be responsible for these eruptions.

The following pages include a discussion of three common forms of contact dermatitis: poison ivy, cosmetic contact dermatitis, and occupational dermatoses. These represent a large percentage of the skin afflictions suffered by the general population. Also included is a section on ear-piercing. The nickel contained in most earrings is a common culprit in contact dematitis.

Poison Ivy Dermatitis

"Leaflets three, let it be" is an old poetic warning. To which let me add my own, unpoetic, "Don't be rash with poison ivy."

The three-leafer is the most common cause of contact dermatitis in the United States. The common poison ivy can be found in every state except California and Nevada. Poison sumac grows primarily along the eastern seaboard. Poison oak grows in California, Oregon, and Washington. The plants can grow as vines attaching themselves to walls, fences, trees, telephone poles, and other vines, or they can be found as ground shrubs of various sizes.

Despite its name, poison ivy is not a poison. And, it is *not* contagious. It is an allergic substance—one that can cause skin rashes in susceptible individuals. A person rubs against or is in some other manner exposed to the poison ivy plant. A certain chemical in the plant acts as a foreign material (antigen) on the skin, thereby stirring up a defensive mechanism in our body. Certain "protective" cells (antibodies) are formed, and the response to the combination of the foreign and protective substances takes the form of redness, blisters, and itching which we know as poison ivy dermatitis.

You can develop a dermatitis from poison ivy by direct contact, such as walking through the woods, indirect contact (from exposure to contaminated shoes and other articles of clothing, sports equipment, and animals which may have run through poison ivy patches), and by burning poison ivy leaves, which can cause reactions on the eyelids and face due to active material in the smoke.

Not all people exposed to the poison ivy plant will develop the rash. If, however, the individual has a history of poison ivy affairs, then the rash will appear within a few hours after exposure. If the person has never had poison ivy dermatitis before, the rash may develop in two to three weeks after the initial exposure.

Poison ivy dermatitis knows no season. More cases, however, occur in late spring and early summer, when the plant sap is most abundant in the stem and leaves.

Although poison ivy dermatitis is not contagious, you yourself can spread the rash to other parts of your body within the first hour after contact. After one hour on the skin, the chemical responsible for the rash will have changed so that no further contamination can occur. However, inanimate objects, such as golf clubs or the clothes you were wearing at the time, can retain the substance for months, thus producing the rash when least expected.

Treatment for poison ivy dermatitis depends upon the severity of the eruption.

In the mild, fairly localized cases, compressing the area with warm water and applying plain calamine lotion (no other fancy, over-the-counter poison ivy remedies are recommended) help dry up the tiny blisters and relieve the itching.

In the more extensive and moderately severe eruptions, it is wise to see your physician. You may need an oral medication in the form of antihistamines for the itching and a possible antibiotic if secondary infection has occurred.

In the really severe cases, where the blisters are huge, the rash has become generalized, and the itching is intense, your doctor may prescribe cortisone-type injections or pills, along with soothing therapeutic baths and creams, to help you over the most uncomfortable phase.

For more treatment information, see page 99.

Cosmetic Contact Dermatitis

In our society many women—and men, too—go to great lengths to look and smell good. This pursuit is reinforced by the countless products on the market that claim to help us retain our youthful, healthy looks.

How many products might you put on your face, hair, body and nails before you leave the house? From the top:

On your hair, you might use conditioner, color or tint, shampoo, creme rinse, setting lotion, and hair spray. Bleach? Hair-straightener? Permanent wave solution? In the bath you might use soap, bath oil, bath oil beads, bath salts, powder, and body lotion. And on your face—for starters—there would be soap or cleansing cream and astringent, perhaps followed by moisturizer, foundation base, tinted base, shading cream, highlighting cream, contour cream, toner, blusher, blotter, face powder, and mineral water spray. Your eyes are next—eye shadow, eye liner, eyebrow pencil, eyebrow powder, and mascara. Eyecircle concealer? False eyelashes and glue? Lash extenders? For the lips—gloss, rouge and lip liner.

Your fingernails and toenails will demand a cuticle cream, base coat, nail conditioner, nail hardener, nail lacquer, nail gloss, and quick-dry solution. Artificial nails, perhaps? And don't forget the depilatory, hygiene spray, deodorant and anti-perspirant, hand cream, and perfume.

Did I forget anything?

Would you believe that each product just mentioned—58 in all—can cause a skin allergy, hair breakage, or nail discoloration? There isn't a product on the market, including even the so-called hypoallergenic varieties that cannot at some time, in some person, produce a contact dermatitis on the skin.

A person may use a cosmetic product for years without developing a reaction and suddenly become allergic to any of a number of substances in the formulation. These substances include chemicals and preservatives, lanolin, dyes, and fragrances.

Dermatitis does not always occur in the area where the cosmetic is applied. Dermatitis of the eyelids or neck, for example, could be due to nail polish or hair spray.

The chief causes of cosmetic dermatitis in men are shave creams (particularly the self-heating types), hair dyes, hair tonics, adhesives for hair pieces, antibacterial soaps, colognes and after-shave lotions, deodorants, sunscreens, and clear nail polish.

How can you tell whether or not you have an allergy to a cosmetic, and what can you do about it? Determine what new products you may have been exposed to just before your rash appeared and then eliminate all possible irritants. Change soaps to a mild, white, perfume-free variety. (Lowila Cake is an excellent soap substitute.) Discontinue all scented lotions, creams, and sprays. Use no cosmetics for a week, then gradually return to them one at a time. Or, better yet, try to live without a lot of them. The fewer the chemicals to which the skin is exposed, the less chance of it being irritated or sensitized.

You should also consider culprits other than what you yourself might be using. Have you been around anyone who wore a new perfume, cologne or other scented toiletries? Anything new at the beauty shop or barber? At work? The possibilities are infinite.

If you cannot pinpoint the cause of your problem, your general physician, allergist, or dermatologist may have the proper knowledge and equipment to determine the cause. And, unless you eliminate the cause, you will forever be plagued with this hypersensitivity rash whenever you are exposed to your nemesis.

Occupational Dermatoses

At last count, there were 90 million people working in more than 55,000 forms of employment—a staggering number of occupations. And any of these 55,000 occupations can be responsible for contact dermatitis and other skin diseases.

The skin has many functions, not the least of which is to protect us from a hostile environment which includes radiation, germs, irritants, blows, chemicals, and temperature changes. Yet despite the ability of this mechanism to withstand many of these onslaughts, the skin is still the most commonly injured organ.

Here are a few facts:

- Skin eruptions account for about 75% of all medical diseases compensated for and are the number one in-plant cause of lost time in industry.
- Fully 10% of all skin diseases in the general population are industrial in origin.
- The cost of skin diseases due to occupational exposure runs into the hundreds of millions of dollars a year in medical expenses and lost time on the job.
- 4 out of 5 cases of occupational contact dermatitis involve only the hands.

Occupational dermatitis is defined as a "contact dermatitis for which exposure at work can be shown to be the main cause or one of the factors contributing to its occurrence." Direct causes of occupational or industrial skin disease can be divided into seven groups:

1. Chemicals, the most frequent cause, include strong acids and alkalis, solvents, cutting oils, gases, and salts. All can injure the skin on direct contact, producing various rashes, while other chemicals, such as those found in leather, lacquer or rubber, can cause rashes which are allergic in nature.
2. Mechanical factors, caused by pressure and friction (for example, prolonged use of pneumatic tools, such as air hammers and chisels), are responsible for cuts, bruises, calluses, and the like. Fiberglas can produce a mechanical irritation and an itchy rash.
3. Physical factors in the form of excessive heat, sunlight, wind, and cold can cause burns, sunburns, allergic reactions, and frostbite.
4. Bacterial and fungal infections can occur among meat handlers, farmers and grocers.
5. Insect bites and stings among outside workers are common dermatologic afflictions.
6. Bites from snakes and wild animals may occur among zookeepers, outdoor workers, garbage men, and mailmen.
7. Vegetation in the form of poisonous plants and woods, causing such skin eruptions as poison ivy, poison oak, and poison sumac dermatitis, can be found among gardeners, farmers, road builders, surveyors, and telephone workers.

There are hundreds of products and chemicals in industry that can cause dermatitis in otherwise healthy people. Almost anything can be responsible, but certain occupations are more susceptible than others to contact dermatitis.

The following are some of the more common occupations and material used in these jobs that are responsible for skin rashes:

Artists: Turpentine, solvents, clay, plaster, paint, sprays, ink.

Auto mechanics: Solvents, cutting oils, paints, cleansers, greases, kerosene, lacquer.

Bakers: Flour, spices, cinnamon, nuts, lemon, flavorings.

Barbers and hairdressers: Soaps, shampoos, permanent-wave solutions, hair dyes, rubber gloves, bleaching agents.

Bartenders: Detergents, cleansers, citrus fruits.

Bookbinders: Glue, plastics, solvents.

Building tradespeople: Cement, epoxy resins, rubber and leather gloves.

Butchers: Detergents, meat.

Canning industry: Juices, dyes, preservatives, brine.

Carpenters: Polishes, glues, solvents, cleansers, adhesives.

Clerks and office workers: Carbon paper, glue, typewriter ribbons, copy paper, rubber, nickel.

Cooks: Meat and vegetable juices, spices, detergents.

Dentists and dental technicians: Resins, acrylics, fluxes, mercury, local anesthetics.

Dry cleaners: Benzene, turpentine, carbon tetrachloride.

Electricians: Rubber, tape, glues, soldering flux, solvents.

Exterminators: Arsenic, DDT, formaldehyde, pyrethrum.

Florists and gardeners: Fertilizer, pesticides, plants (tulips, chrysanthemums, narcissus).

Food industry: Detergents, vegetables, spices, rubber gloves.

Foundry work: Oils, hand cleansers, resins, plastics.

Garment and millinery industries: Dyes, turpentine, benzene.

Groceries and delicatessen: Dyes on labels, insecticides, cardboard boxes, paper bags.

Hospital workers: Soaps, detergents, disinfectants, rubber gloves, penicillin, streptomycin.

Household workers: Detergents, polishes, solvents, rubber gloves, sprays.

Jewelers: Solvents, nickel, enamels, chrome.

Laundry workers: Detergents, bleaches, solvents, turpentine, starch, antiseptics, soaps.

Manicurists: Nail polish, acrylic plastic (nails), cosmetics.

Masons: Cement, acids, resins, rubber and leather gloves.

Medical technicians and nurses: Detergents, solvents, plastics, antibiotics, antiseptics, anesthetics, formalin, rubber gloves.

Metal workers: Cutting oils, cleansers, solvents.

Painters: Turpentine, thinners, solvents, paints, dyes and adhesives in wallpaper.

Paper manufacturers: Glues and pastes.

Photographers: Acids, solvents, formaldehyde, dyes, color developers.

Plastic industry: Solvents, acids, additives, hardeners.

Platers: Solvents, paints, chromium, acids and alkalis.

Plumbers: Oils, hand cleansers, rubber, cement, nickel.

Printers: Solvents, glues, turpentine, paper finishes.

Rubber workers: Solvents, rubber, dyes, tars.

Shoemakers: Solvents, glues, leather, rubber, turpentine, cement, polishes.

Sporting goods: Lead, rubber, nickel, chrome, leather, dyes.

Textile workers: Solvents, bleaching agents, fibers, dyes, finishes.

Theatrical profession: Cosmetics, dyes, woods.

Undertakers: Formaldehyde, embalming fluids.

Welders: Oil, chromium, nickel.

Window shade makers: Paint, benzene, shellac.

Woodworkers: Woods, turpentine, lacquers, varnish, tars, paints.

What is particularly sobering is that fully *90 percent* of all occupational dermatoses can be controlled and prevented by protective clothing and cleansers.

The cure of contact dermatitis depends largely on detection and removal of the cause. This search for the causes can be one of the most intricate tasks confronting an allergist or dermatologist. But once the causative agent has been discovered, it is relatively simple to cure the skin rash and prevent recurrences.

Treating Contact Dermatitis

The specific treatment for contact dermatitis due to chemicals, plants (such as poison ivy), cosmetics, metals, irritant substances, etc. is essentially the same as for the treatment of eczema.

Compresses

For the acute, localized contact dermatitis, as found in poison ivy or nail polish dermatitis, use warm compresses with any of the following:

AluWets Wet Dressing Crystals (Stiefel)

Directions: Dissolve contents of one packet in 12 ounces of warm water and apply as open wet dressings for 15 to 20 minutes every hour or two.

Domeboro Powder Packets (Dome)

Directions: Dissolve contents of one packet in a pint (16 ounces) of warm water and apply as above.

Bluboro Powder (Herbert)

Directions: Dissove contents of one packet in a pint (16 ounces) of warm water and apply as above.

Baths

For widespread areas of contact dermatitis, soothing baths in any of the following often give prompt relief of the symptoms:

Alpha Keri Therapeutic Bath Oil (Westwood)
nutraSpa Bath Oil (Owen)
Aveeno Oilated Bath (Cooper)

Directions for all of the above: Follow the directions provided on the containers.

Creams & Lotions

When the acute phase of the dermatitis has begun to clear, discontinue the wet dressings and the baths. Apply a lotion or cream to help relieve the itching and restore the skin to its normal color and texture. Use either of the following compounded preparations:

Phenol	**½%**
Calamine Lotion (USP)	**to make 4 oz.**

or

Menthol	**¼%**
Phenol	**½%**
Cold Cream	**to make 2 oz.**

Or use the following over-the-counter preparations:

Rhulicort Cream (Lederle)
Rhulicort Lotion (Lederle)
Schamberg's Lotion (C & M Pharmacal)

Directions for all of the above: Apply to the affected areas every 3 or 4 hours.

Soap Substitutes

Never use soaps on the affected areas of contact dermatitis. Only the following soap substitutes may be used for cleansing purposes:

Lowila Cake (Westwood)
Aveenobar (Cooper)

Oral Medications

For the itching that usually accompanies every phase of contact dermatitis, take the following antihistamine every 4 hours whenever necessary:

Chlor-Trimeton Tablets 4 mg (Schering)

And, above all, avoid the particular agent that started the dermatitis in the first place!

Ear-Piercing

'Ear ye! 'Ear ye! Pierced ears are back in vogue, and many teen-agers, as well as adult women, are having it done.

And one of the latest fads—eerie, in a way—is that some women are having each ear pierced in three or four different places and wear as many as six or eight earrings at one time.

It may come as a surprise to many, but pierced earrings were common ornaments of men in England up to the 17th century. The custom was common in the British Navy up to the mid-19th century. It was widespread in some of the Balkan subcultures up until World War I. And it was common in the U.S. Navy up to about 50 years ago! There has been a recent revival of this custom in young men who wear single earrings in their left ears.

Yet, harmless as the custom may seem, it isn't something that should be done casually by friends, relatives, or other unskilled individuals.

The ear-piercing procedure itself takes only a few moments, is relatively painless, and is best performed by a physician who is aware of proper sterile technique as well as some of the minor hazards that may accompany it. The medical societies in many states consider ear-piercing a surgical procedure and a part of the practice of medicine. It is illegal in these states for anyone, except a physician, to pierce ears.

People with certain diseases should not have their ears pierced. They include those with a history of eczema, diabetes, rheumatic fever, certain blood disorders, impetigo, the cystic type of acne, and allergies to metals.

The American Medical Association has recently warned the public of some of the complications of ear-piercings, particularly when done under unsterile conditions: hepatitis and other internal infections (in rare cases leading to death); excessive bleeding which may form a blood tumor (hematoma); raised scars, or keloids, which can occur in susceptible people; and allergic sensitization to the metal (usually nickel) in the earrings.

Many earrings today, particularly the cheaper varieties, contain nickel. Nickel is a powerful sensitizer, especially in contact with broken skin. And so, lately, there has been a "rash" of skin allergies on earlobes which resemble infection. For the most part this reaction is merely an inflammation. Occasionally, however, certain bacteria take up housekeeping on the raw, broken skin, resulting in a true infection with weeping, oozing, and crusting. If this occurs, you must consult a physician.

To prevent this type of allergic phenomenon, purchase trainer earrings made of surgical stainless steel. In addition to being made of stainless steel, these trainer earrings (which can be quite elaborate depending upon the place of purchase) should be of the "post" type. Hoops and wires are not recommended until at least three months after the ear-piercing procedure. One company that has a line of allergy-free earrings is H & A Enterprises, 143-19 25th Avenue, Whitestone, New York 11357. Write them and ask for their catalogue.

Should you have it done? If you are healthy, if you plan to have your ears pierced in a clean and sterile manner by a physician, if you do not have a history of being allergic to metals, and if you have no raised scars on your skin, the chances are that you will have no complications following your ear-piercing.

Here are some other hints to help prevent infection:

- After having your ears pierced, wear the same earrings continuously for at least 6 weeks.

- Gently wash the front and back of your earlobes with soap and water at least twice daily. (Do not use alcohol to clean these areas, as the alcohol may dissolve or in some way react with the glue that cements the ball to the post.)
- Twirl (turn) the earrings several complete revolutions 2 or 3 times daily.
- Some amount of redness and tenderness is normal after ear-piercing. If any unusual pain, swelling, or discharge develops, contact the physician who did the procedure.

4 Tumors of the Skin

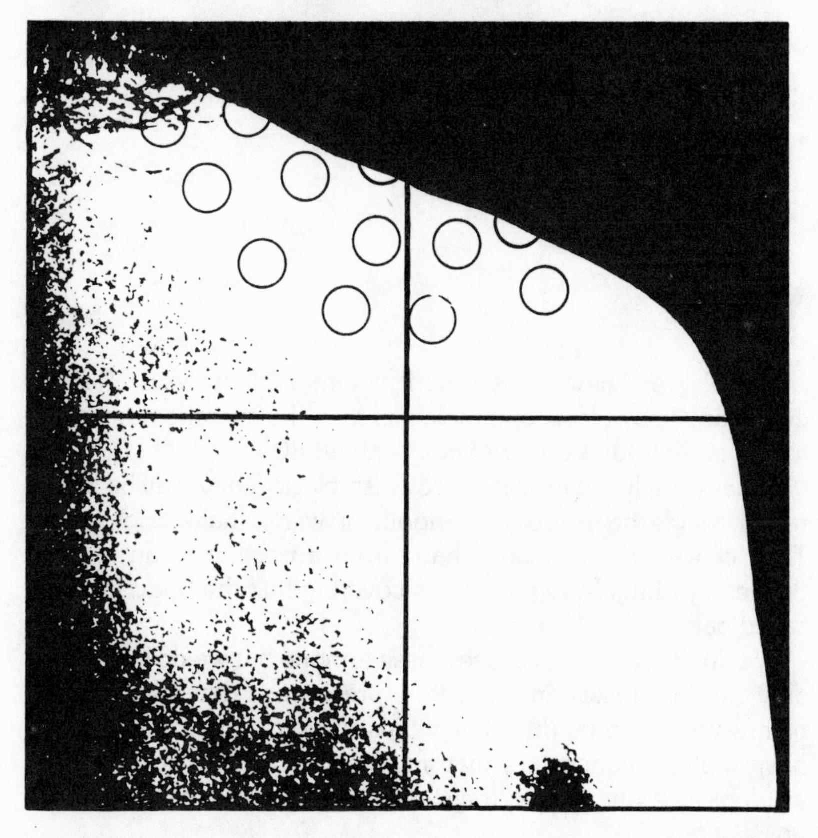

A tumor is a swelling or new growth.

Tumors, which are mistakenly thought to be only malignant, include a wide variety of growths, both benign (friendly) or malignant (unfriendly), that can affect any organ of the body. Benign skin tumors include warts, moles, molluscums, seborrheic keratoses, and skin tags. Common malignant skin tumors include the epitheliomas (carcinomas) and the malignant melanoma.

Almost every person will develop some type of skin tumor in his or her lifetime, but the great majority of skin tumors are benign, of little consequence, and never brought to the attention of the physician.

Moles

A mole, or "nevus," is a benign tumor of the skin. Almost everybody has at least one mole—in fact, the average number of moles on the adult human body is about 40.

Moles usually are brown or brownish-black. They may be flat or raised, single or in groups, smooth or warty, hairless or hairy. They can vary in size and shape from a fraction of an inch in diameter to huge, irregular areas covering half the body (the so-called bathing-trunk nevus).

We don't know what causes these tumors, but we do know that they run in families and that their presence is determined even before you're born. (In other words, if your father and mother have moles, chances are that you will, too.) What these moles will look like and where they'll occur, however, seems to be a quirk of fate.

Moles which appear at birth often are called, quite appropriately, "birthmarks." The so-called "strawberry mark" (known medically as a hemangioma) is one of the most common. It manifests itself as a blood blister of varying size and may appear almost anywhere on the body. Another common type of birthmark is the port-wine stain (nevus flammeus), a flat, reddish-purple mark which is seen most often on the back of the neck and the face. Some birthmarks fade after 3 or 4 years; others last a lifetime.

Most moles, however, don't develop until puberty or

adolescence. They grow rapidly over a period of years and then slowly disappear—as if fading into the skin—in old age. Surprisingly, people in their 70s and 80s have very few moles.

The fashionable mole of famous women of a bygone era was a fortuitous happenstance. Strategically placed on a woman's cheek, it was considered a sign of beauty, and the name "beauty mark" still is used in many households. Jean Harlow and Marilyn Monroe had moles. Elizabeth Taylor and Telly Savalas have moles.

Other people, however, don't share this admiration for their own moles and seek to have them removed. The usual method for removing small moles is surgical excision under local anesthesia, a relatively simple office procedure.

Although moles are harmless, they may change and become darker, causing concern. This can be due to exposure to the sun and to certain types of medications, such as cortisone. Hormone changes during puberty and pregnancy also may cause moles to become larger and darker and may even cause new ones to appear. Generally, these changes are no cause for alarm. On rare occasions, however, changes in a mole can indicate a melanoma, the dreaded "black cancer." Although one of the most dangerous and fatal of all cancers, melanomas have an excellent cure rate if recognized early and followed by complete and wide excision.

So, if your mole suddenly becomes larger or darker, bleeds or crusts, or becomes itchy or painful, consult your physician at once. Your doctor may recommend that the tumor be completely excised or may opt to remove surgically a small piece of tissue (known as a biopsy) and have it examined microscopically to determine the nature and extent of the apparent change. Most likely, your lesion will prove to be benign, but only a doctor can give you this reassurance.

Keratoses

Keratoses are tumors of the skin that occur in most individuals in the latter decades of life.

There are two kinds of keratoses, the most common being the harmless seborrheic keratoses. These are greasy, light-brown, slightly raised growths that chiefly involve the face, chest, and back. They are slow-growing, loosely attached to the skin, and are usually covered by a waxy crust. They may be single or multiple and are usually round or oval, although they may be seen in any shape. They vary in size from a fraction of an inch in diameter up to half-dollar size or larger.

Many people are fond of scraping them off with their fingernails—a habit that is not recommended. They may become infected, and they invariably grow back if not completely removed.

Seborrheic keratoses appear to run in families. They become more numerous with advancing age, and are not infectious or contagious. Also, fortunately, they never become malignant (cancerous).

Senile keratoses (also called solar or actinic keratoses), on the other hand, are very early skin cancers. And the culprit in all cases is the sun.

Localized primarily over the sun-exposed portions of the body—face, ears, forearms and backs of hands—they are commonly seen in people frequently exposed to the sun: the farmer, the sailor, the fisherman, the cattleman.

These tumors are rough, dry, reddish-brown, dirty-looking growths that are firmly planted in the skin surface. If not treated, some of these may, after many years, undergo serious malignant degeneration, in other words, become cancerous. When this happens, there is the danger of the condition spreading to lymph glands and internal organs.

There are no internal remedies for seborrheic keratoses—either curative or preventive—and no salves or ointments that will rid a person of these "barnacles of old age." For cosmetic reasons, and (in the case of the more sinister senile keratoses) for medical reasons, some people choose to have them removed.

Your physician can remove them by any of the following methods:

- *Electrosurgery.* After the lesion has been anesthetized, it is burned with the electric current and then scraped off with a round knife (dermal curette). Post-operative bleeding is minimal, and the entire procedure takes only a few minutes.
- *Curettage.* Following a local anesthetic, the lesion is scraped off in the same manner as described above, except there is no burning. (Very small lesions may be destroyed by this method even without the use of anesthesia, but this method is usually reserved for stoics.)
- *Liquid nitrogen therapy.* This extremely cold substance (minus 320° F) is applied to the keratoses for a few seconds by means of a cotton applicator or a spray-type device. Over the next few days, the areas blister and the lesions are pushed out. There is only minimal discomfort, and the cosmetic results are excellent.

A physician can treat a dozen or more of these tumors by these methods (depending upon the size and location) without great inconvenience to the patient.

In addition, there is a chemical substance (5 FU) which, when locally applied, selectively picks out the "disagreeable" cells of senile keratoses. The chemical creates a moderately severe reaction in the skin for a few weeks. Then, after the process has reached its peak, the area slowly heals. It leaves the skin smooth and supple, with no scarring. This method is recommended for multiple senile keratoses, particularly those about the face and scalp.

For those with a tendency to develop senile keratoses, it is extremely important to avoid the sun. If your occupation requires sun exposure, the use of a protective sunscreen, such as PreSun, is a must.

Only your physician can treat your keratoses. However, to prevent the precancerous, actinic keratoses from forming, always use a sun-protective agent such as those listed on page 125.

Skin Cancer

Malignant tumors of the skin are the most common cancers of the human body. They're also the easiest forms of malignancy to treat. Almost 100% of all skin cancers are completely curable.

Since the skin is the largest and most exposed organ of the body, it is vulnerable to more environmental attacks from injury, weather, and sunlight than other organs. This, as well as exposure of the skin to certain chemicals and industrial compounds, such as tar and arsenic, predispose our large "envelope" to malignant growths.

While the cause of skin cancer, like all cancers, remains a mystery, we do know a fair amount about the nature of the disease. Cancer of the skin occurs most frequently in fair-haired people—those who lack sufficient quantities of melanin, a pigment substance that filters out the harmful rays of the sun. It is a common disease of farmers, sailors, fishermen and athletes who often spend a lifetime outdoors.

There are two common types of skin malignancies: basal cell carcinoma and squamous cell carcinoma.

The basal cell carcinoma, the least aggressive of all cancers of the skin, grows very slowly and almost never spreads to distant areas of the body. It is characterized by a pearly, waxy-looking nodule which may ulcerate after a period of time. It is a "friendly" malignancy and is completely curable if removed before extensive growth has occurred. When left untreated, these slow-growing tumors invade and destroy the adjacent and deeper tissues. But they almost never metastasize (spread) to internal organs.

The squamous cell carcinoma, on the other hand, is a relatively dangerous tumor, one which, if allowed to grow, can spread to involve the nearby lymph glands and internal organs. Fortunately, these cancers, which occur primarily on the sun-exposed areas of the face, ears, neck and hands, are much rarer than the basal cell type.

Early recognition and prompt, adequate treatment for all malignancies of the skin are essential. Early signs include any new growth that does not heal or any *change* in an existing growth. If you have either of these symptoms, see your physician at once.

If "unfriendly" cells are suspected, your doctor will surgically remove a small piece of diseased tissue and have it examined microscopically for any possibility of malignancy. This procedure is known as a biopsy. If the tumor is malignant, the treatment will depend upon the location and size of the growth, the nature of the cancerous cells, and whether or not any spread is evident. For the small, simple, "friendly" basal cell cancers, cauterization with the electric needle or surgical removal are quick, simple and safe procedures which can be performed in the doctor's office. Other methods include freezing techniques, locally-applied chemicals which selectively eradicate the malignant cells, and X-ray therapy. Regardless of the type of therapy, healing is a slow process and scarring is an inevitable consequence.

In all cases and by whatever means, complete destruction or removal of the entire tumor must be accomplished. Periodic follow-up by your physician is necessary to insure against any recurrence of the lesion.

To prevent skin cancers, fair-haired and sun-sensitive people should avoid excessive sun exposure. At the same time, *everyone* should wear protective clothing (wide-brimmed hats, gloves and long sleeves) and use commercial sun-screen lotions to filter out the harmful and cancer-producing rays of the sun.

Melanoma

Evidence from many sources suggests a steadily rising incidence of melanoma in the past few decades accompanied by a rising death rate. It accounts for most of the deaths from skin cancer. The mortality rate in the United States from this deadly tumor is now about 3,000 per year.

What is this malignant growth that seems to appear suddenly out of nowhere and quickly invades not only adjacent tissue but distant organs, spreading via the blood and lymph channels?

Malignant melanomas are usually black lesions of the skin which arise in a pre-existing, dark, hairless mole—hence the epithet "black cancer." They can also be pale and non-pigmented. While occurring mainly on the skin surface, melanomas can appear in the eye, on mucous membranes, and elsewhere. No portion of the body and no organ is immune from this lethal tumor. It can occur at any age but is seen most commonly in people between 40 and 70.

No single cause for melanoma has been discovered, but some of the following factors appear to be involved:

- There is a higher incidence of malignant melanoma in summer climates. The incidence in Australia is 17/100,000; in Connecticut, 4/100,000; and in Scotland, 2.3/100,000.
- There is a higher incidence in whites due to the superior ultraviolet screening capacity provided by black skin.

- People who develop melanoma are likely to have light-colored eyes, light complexions, light hair-color and are inclined to sunburn rather easily.
- While melanomas are uncommon in blacks, they can occur on the more lightly pigmented portions of the skin: the palms, soles, and mucous membranes of the mouth.
- More melanomas develop on the legs of women than men. This is thought to be due to greater exposure to sunlight due to women's habit of dress.
- It has also been suggested that women taking birth control pills run a far greater risk of developing these black cancers than those women who have never been on the oral contraceptives.
- Injury may also play a role in the development of melanoma. In the barefooted African Bantu, melanoma of the sole is higher than in those who wear shoes; and in Ugandans the most common site of melanoma is on the sole.

Bleak as this picture is, melanoma can be cured surgically in over 50 percent of cases. The key to success is prompt therapy. One can never be certain, however, that a malignant melanoma has actually been cured, particularly those tumors that are of the deeper variety—those that have entered the lower layers of the skin and subcutaneous tissue and have spread to involve the lymph glands.

How do you know whether or not to worry about existing moles? A mole undergoing any growth or any change in size, contour or color should be suspect. Moles that bleed or ulcerate also point to malignant change. See your physician at once if you notice any of these changes. He or she will more than likely recommend surgical excision of the worrisome mole followed by microscopic analysis of the tissue.

Molluscum Contagiosum

Unlike the skin tumors discussed so far, a molluscum is caused by a virus, the largest of all true viruses known to cause human disease. Sometimes referred to as a "dimple wart," this common, benign tumor appears most frequently in children and young adults.

Molluscums are contagious—thus, the term, molluscum contagiosum. They can spread indirectly (through towels, washcloths, and the like) or directly from person to person. Epidemics of these virus tumors are common among children in schools, orphanages, and other institutions.

It usually takes about six weeks from the time of contact or exposure to the virus until the disease becomes manifest. It enters the skin through small injuries (scratches, insect bites, puncture wounds, etc.). The molluscums usually begin as pin-head sized elevations which gradually enlarge to the size of a small pea. They may persist for years but usually stop growing once they reach this size.

The elevations—known as nodules—are smooth, round, dome-shaped, and either waxy or pearly in appearance. On the surface of the mature lesion is usually a dimple, or "umbilication" (resembling a belly-button). They neither itch, hurt, nor burn. When squeezed, they discharge a milky-white, curd-like substance.

Left untreated, the lesions usually disappear by themselves

after months or years without leaving scars. Since they are contagious, however, there are some measures you should take.

To prevent the spread of the condition, avoid direct contact with known infected people and practice good hygiene (keep clean!). Your physician also can eradicate them quickly and almost painlessly by any of a variety of methods. One popular method is to freeze them off with liquid nitrogen (minus 320°F). They can also be burned off, or cauterized, under local anesthesia, scraped off with a small curette (actually a "round knife"), or destroyed with various chemicals. All of these methods are safe and effective.

Treating Molluscum Contagiosum

Since molluscums are viral tumors, it is often difficult to rid yourself of them with anything except surgical or freezing techniques used by the physician. The following preparations, however, procured from your pharmacist, may help destroy early, small lesions:

Local Medications

5% Ammoniated Mercury Ointment
(Lilly)

Directions: Gently rub into each lesion twice daily using a cotton-tipped applicator.

This preparation has to be compounded by your pharmacist. Ask that it be put it in a glass-rod applicator bottle.

Salicylic acid	**5%**
Lactic acid	**5%**
Flexible Collodion	**to make ½ oz.**

Directions: Apply to the tops of each lesion at bedtime.

If, after 2 or 3 weeks, the lesions show no sign of budging, or if new lesions have appeared, see your physician.

5 Sun-Related Skin Conditions

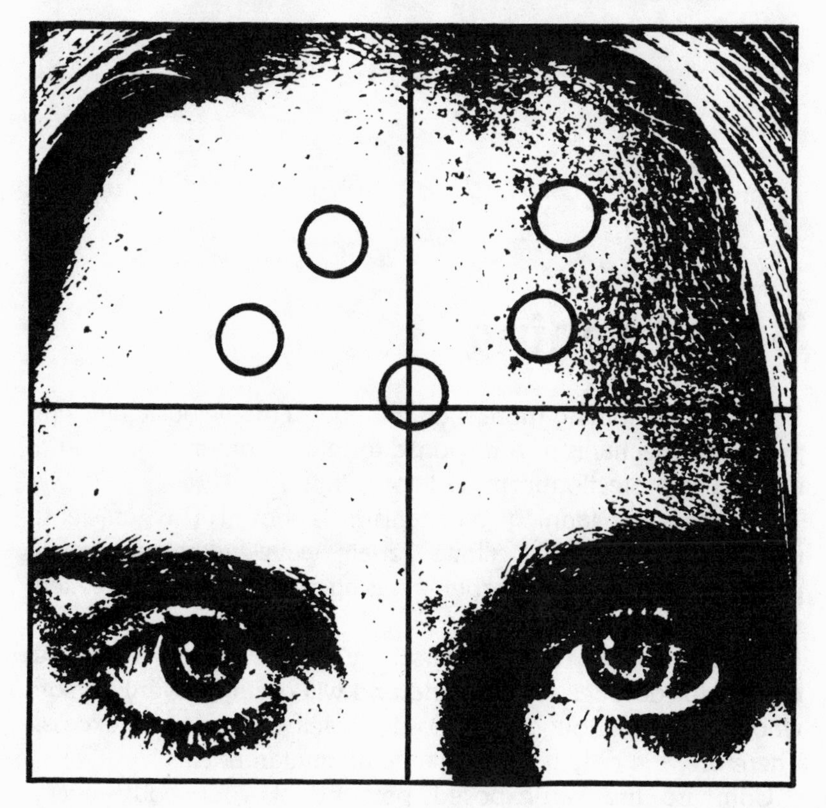

The suntan. The envy of friends and relatives. The bronzed lifeguard; the golden, tawny bodies on the sand.

The sad truth is that sun-tanning is a dangerous habit with no benefit except the elusive psychological one: looking good and healthy means feeling good and healthy. Exposure to the sun is directly and ultimately responsible for the leathery look of prematurely aged skin, wrinkles, and skin cancer—all of which are irreversible. It can also cause sun-poisoning.

Skin cancer was discussed in Chapter 4. The following sections describe the process behind sun-tanning, how to sun-tan properly, and how to treat and prevent sun-poisoning.

Sun-Tanning

Tanning is nothing more than the body's marvelously efficient protective mechanism: a response to injury from sunlight and a method of protection from additional injury.

Because the tanning mechanism is not 100% efficient, repeated sun exposure allows certain wavelengths of light to penetrate this defense barrier, causing the various sun-related skin conditions.

The more subtle changes caused by the sun's rays may not be evident for decades, but they do and will occur in every person who is foolish enough to expose himself or herself to excess. Therefore, the only good suntan is no suntan at all.

Compare the sun-exposed portions of your body—face, hands, forearms—with those parts of your anatomy (your buttocks, for example) that are almost never exposed. Note the difference in smoothness and texture. Your buttocks are young; your hands and face are old.

For fair-haired, fair-skinned, and blue-eyed people, tanning, if it does occur, is a slow process. They have far less pigment cells than their dark-haired, darker-skinned, brown-eyed neighbors. So they burn more readily and require infinitely more sun exposure to produce even a modest tan. In darker-skinned people, on the other hand, merely a brief exposure to the sun often produces a lasting tan.

For those light-skinned people who, despite all admonition,

still desire the bronzed look, here are a few rules:

Acquire your tan gradually. If you head for the beaches, the backyards, and the lake in order to soak up that first Sunday sun in June, avoid a severe, painful, disfiguring sunburn accompanied by swelling and blisters by limiting the first exposure to 15 or 20 minutes. Increase the exposure gradually by 20 or 30 minutes per day for 4 or 5 more days at which time the first pigment cells will begin to show up to darken and protect the skin. From then on, almost any length of exposure may be tolerated.

Redheads and blondes, who do not have adequate pigment cells to begin with, must be more careful and reduce the early exposure times by approximately half.

All this, however, is trial and error. Only *you* will know how much sun you can tolerate on first and subsequent exposures without causing painful sunburn.

Keep in mind that the most intense rays of the sun occur between 10 a.m. and 2 p.m. (standard time), the overhead sun being the strongest. You cannot get sunburned before 9 a.m. and after 5 p.m., at which times the sharply angulated "burn" rays have been filtered out by the atmosphere.

Also, don't be fooled by overcast skies: sunburn can occur on hazy and foggy days. And don't think that only direct exposure to the sun produces burning or tanning. Reflected rays from sand, cement, and water can also cause severe sunburn. Even beach umbrellas do not offer absolute protection.

Use suntan creams and lotions. Many of the suntan preparations that can be purchased in the drugstore contain certain chemicals which selectively absorb the shorter wavelengths of sunlight that are responsible for burning. This will permit some of the longer wavelengths—the tanning rays—to penetrate the skin and allow the desirable tanning results.

People have been classified into various skin types depending upon their levels of melanin pigmentation. And, depending upon the type of skin you have, there is a wide range of sunscreen products that have been rated according to the degree of protection they can give against ultraviolet radiation. This rating is known as the Sun Protection Factor (SPF). A list of these products, with the appropriate SPF, appears on page 125.

Skin Type I: People with fair skin and fair hair or freckles are most susceptible to the sun's rays. They can develop a severe sunburn in a matter of minutes and also have a higher risk of developing skin cancers and wrinkles.These people are advised to use sunscreens with a Sun Protection Factor of 10-15.

Skin Type II: These people are also fair-skinned but not as sensitive to the sun's rays as those of Type I. They ususally burn and only occasionally develop a "weak" tan. These people are advised to use suncreens with a Sun Protection Factor of 6-10.

(Types I and II comprise about one-third of the population. People with these skin types should not try to acquire a tan.)

Skin Type III: This type includes people with darker skin who usually tan but sometimes burn. These people are advised to use sunscreens with an SPF of 4-6.

Skin Type IV: These people always tan well and almost never develop sunburn. They can use sunscreens with an SPF of 2-4.

When using any sun-tanning product, follow the directions given by the manufacturer, and re-apply it every 2 or 3 hours. Always re-apply after swimming.

The best approach to sun-tanning is common sense. This large envelope we call the skin has to last a lifetime, so give it the protection it deserves.

A word about those new tanning salons that are springing up all over the country. The ultraviolet tanning lamps used in these salons are fraught with the same hazards as other forms of radiation. There are definite dangers associated with repeated exposure to these ultraviolet lamps. They include skin damage in the form of premature aging, wrinkles, senile keratoses, and cancer of the skin. Forewarned, forearmed!

Sun-Poisoning

Sun-poisoning is a non-scientific term referring to several abnormal responses to the rays of the sun which occur in certain people often in combination with a variety of drugs, chemicals, cosmetics, and plants. It can occur in anyone who is exposed to enough light (which reacts with certain chemicals in the skin), or has insufficient protective skin pigment, or both.

The classic example of sun-poisoning is sunburn. We all know that redheads suffer more from the effects of the sun's rays than the rest of the population. This is because they lack sufficient pigment in the skin—one of the main defenses against sunburn. The black person rarely suffers from sunburn because the pigment present in the epidermis (the upper layers of the skin) prevents the penetration of the sunburn rays into the sensitive layers of the skin.

In susceptible people, certain common drugs taken orally can change the normal protective response to the sun and cause severe rash with blisters on even the slightest exposure to sunlight or fluorescent lighting. Drugs most commonly involved in this type of reaction are the sulfa drugs, "relatives" of tetracycline, various tranquilizers (Thorazine, Compazine and Stelazine), certain high blood pressure medications (Diuril, HydroDIURIL, Esidrix, etc.), and the newer type oral medications for diabetes (Orinase, Diabinese) and fungous infections (griseofulvin).

Sun-poisoning can also occur with exposure to the sun's rays after contact with certain chemicals. The most common substances that cause these "sun-allergic" responses are found in deodorant bar soaps, detergents, certain suntan lotions, shampoos, "first-aid" creams, and various cosmetics and toiletries. One of the greatest offenders is a substance called bithionol, a potent antiseptic which is still used in dozens of soaps and shampoos and various cosmetics.

Even chemicals found in certain vegetables and fruits can cause sun-sensitive eruptions. Gardeners and farmers who, while exposed to the sun, handle such foods as carrots, celery, parsnips, and limes are especially susceptible.

The symptoms of sun allergy consist of severe itching and rash which occur a few days after the combination of the chemical substance and the light. This sensitivity can be so pronounced that a minute amount of the substance left on the skin, followed by exposure even to fluorescent light, may trigger a reaction.

Treatment for sun-poisoning is essentially the same as for any allergic dermatitis, such as poison ivy. If the case is mild, use wet compresses or soothing baths followed by calamine lotion to relieve your symptoms. If the itching is more severe, you may want to take an antihistamine. For severe reactions, accompanied by intense itching and blisters that weep and ooze, see your physician. You may need treatment for dehydration and possible infection.

Prevention of Sun-Poisoning

Preventing sun-sensitive reactions requires trial and error to determine the causative drug, chemical, or plant. Once you have discovered it, eliminate it from your regimen. If the culprit is a drug which is essential for your health (high blood pressure pills, anti-diabetic medication, etc.), it is essential that you stay out of the sun at all times.

If you are fair-skinned, the best way to avoid a sun-sensitive reaction is to stay out of the sun. If this just isn't possible, then tan cautiously, following the guidelines described in the last chapter.

Preventing Sun-Poisoning

To prevent overexposure to the sun, use a good sunscreen. According to the manufacturers, these products contain chemicals which selectively block out or absorb all the harmful, "short" ultraviolet rays, permitting the longer, tanning rays to get through to the skin.

Sunscreens

The following is an accurate sunscreen guide for your skin:

For Skin Type 1—SPF 10-15

PreSun 15 (Westwood)
Total Eclipse (Herbert)
Super Shade (Plough)
Pabanol (Elder)
Solbar Plus 15 (Persōn & Covey)

For Skin Type II—SPF 6-10

PreSun 8 (Westwood)
Eclipse (Herbert)

For Skin Type III—SPF 4-6

PreSun 4 (Westwood)
Partial Eclipse (Herbert)
Solbar (Persōn & Covey)
Sundown (Johnson & Johnson)

For Skin Type IV—SPF 2-4

Sundare (Cooper)
RVP (Elder)

Sunblocks

Another good sun-blocking agent is **zinc oxide paste**. This inexpensive, although cosmetically inelegant, sun-blocking preparation blocks out all the harmful rays of the sun.

To protect the delicate area of the lips, use a "lipstick" that contains sun-blocking agents:

PreSun Sunscreen Lip Protection (Westwood)
Eclipse Sunscreen Lip and Face Protectant (Herbert)
Sun Stick (Cooper)
RVPaba Lipstick (Elder)

Treating Sun-Poisoning

For an acute case of sun-poisoning with redness, itching, burning, and blisters, follow the same treatment you would for the acute contact dermatitis (see pages 99-100).

Compresses

If the condition is localized, use warm, wet compresses with any of the following to allay the itching, burning, blisters, and swelling.

AluWets Wet Dressing Crystals (Stiefel)

Directions: Dissolve contents of one packet in 12 ounces of warm water and apply as open wet dressings for 15 to 20 minutes every hour or two.

Bluboro Powder (Herbert)

Directions: Dissolve contents of one packet in a pint (16 ounces) of warm water and apply as above.

Domeboro Powder Packets (Dome)

Directions: Dissolve contents of one packet in a pint (16 ounces) of warm water and apply as above.

Baths

If the condition is widespread or generalized, take soothing baths in any of the following:

Alpha Keri Therapeutic Bath Oil (Westwood)
nutraSpa Bath Oil (Owen)
Aveeno Oilated Bath (Cooper)

Directions: Follow directions on each container.

A good point to remember is that sun-poisoning is similar to a burn—a fire. Just as you would use water to put out a fire, use wet dressings or baths to relieve a case of sun-poisoning. Never use soap during this phase.

Creams & Lotions

When the acute phase has been relieved, use an emollient cream or lotion to relieve the dryness and flaking that ensues. Try one of the following:

Keri Lotion (Westwood)
Lubriderm Lotion (Parke-Davis)
Neutrogena Lotion (Neutrogena)
Nivea Creme Lotion (Beiersdorf)
Nutraderm Lotion (Owen)
Rhulicort Lotion (Lederle)

Oral Medication

For persistent itching, take the following antihistamine:

Chlor-Trimeton Tablets 4 mg (Schering)

Directions: Take one tablet every four hours when needed for itching.

If the sun-poisoning is severe, with a great deal of pain, huge blisters, or denuded skin, see your physician at once.

To protect from further bouts of sun-poisoning, always use a sunlight protective agent, such as those described above, *before* exposure to the sun.

6 Other Common Skin Afflictions

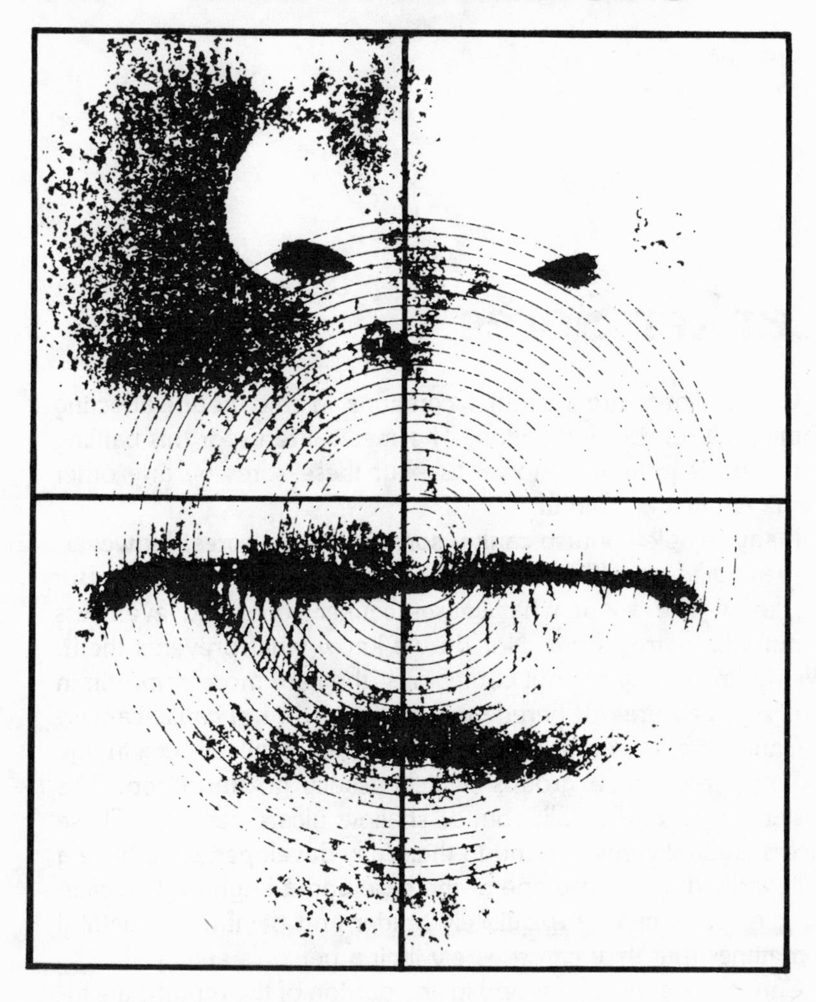

We have already focused on the most common skin conditions. There are, however, literally hundreds more. Other familiar and annoying ailments of the skin and mucous membranes are discussed in the following sections.

Canker Sores

Canker sores are painful ulcerations in the mouth affecting some 25% of the population. The medical term for this baffling condition is aphthous stomatitis—but these sores by any other name are just as painful.

Many people confuse canker sores with cold sores. However, they are different afflictions. Cold sores are caused by a virus. But we know little about what causes canker sores and even less about what cures them. Nor do we know what prevents them. We do know they are not contagious, they are more common in women, they are not hereditary, and they do not cause cancer.

Canker sores, or aphthae, start off as small blisters in the mouth, singly or in groups, which usually go unnoticed. The blisters break and small, round, shallow ulcers develop. These ulcers gradually enlarge and in their fully developed state have a yellowish, shiny membrane at the base and a bright-red swollen margin. They can be exquisitely tender and painful—so painful sometimes that they can severely limit a person's eating.

Canker sores may be found in any portion of the mouth: the inside of the cheeks, the lips, the sides of the tongue, the floor of the mouth, the gums, and the palate. They heal by themselves in about 10 to 14 days without leaving scars. Unfortunately, however, they tend to recur. Some people develop them every few weeks, others every few months, and some unlucky few are never without them.

Although no one knows what causes these painful mouth sores, many of the following triggering factors have been suspected:

- Poor dental hygiene.
- Foods: chocolate, citrus fruits, spices, milk, cola drinks.
- Allergies to drugs or denture materials.
- Illness accompanied by fever.
- Menstruation.
- Fatigue.
- Emotional stress and tension.
- Injury caused by stiff toothbrushes.
- Viruses (similar to the viral infection responsible for cold sores).
- Bacteria.

The latest and most fashionable theory is that canker sores are due to an "autoimmune response." This simply means that there is a self-destructive process going on in the body that is caused by an allergy or sensitivity to one's own tissue. But the fact that there are so many theories—none of which has been substantiated—is reason enough to be certain that no one is actually sure.

What should you do if you have recurrent canker sores? First, see your physician or dentist. Either one may be able to discover a possible reason why you develop these painful and annoying ulcers. Some general measures they might suggest to prevent attacks are the following:

- Keep your mouth clean.
- Eliminate ill-fitting dentures.
- Avoid those foods which you suspect might be a triggering factor.
- Discontinue chewing gum, lozenges, mouthwashes, and menthol cigarettes.
- If you are using a fluoridated toothpaste, change to a nonfluoridated brand or use salt or baking soda as a substitute.
- If they appear before the menstrual period, take an antihistamine daily, beginning a week or 10 days before.

Theories on treating an existing bout of canker sores are almost as varied as the suspected causes. They include numerous folklore remedies, for example, "Chew a small twig from a cherry tree and let the bruised bark rest on the sore spot." Like the treatment of warts, however, these remedies merely attest to the fact that no one really knows what works and how.

Among the many more "scientific" methods are dental ointments containing a "relative" of cortisone, painting the sores with a silver nitrate solution, and using lozenges of one kind or another.

In my opinion, however, there is only one good, proven reliable method: using mouthwashes or compresses that have tetracycline. Tetracycline is a prescription antibiotic and must be ordered by your doctor. This treatment involves emptying a 250-milligram capsule of tetracycline into one ounce of warm water and shaking it up very well. (Tetracycline powder cannot be dissolved in water but forms a suspension when shaken.) You then swish this solution around in your mouth for 5 or 10 minutes every 2 or 3 hours. Or, some physicians will recommend soaking wads of cotton in this suspension and then applying it to the sores. Both methods should give immediate relief.

Treating Canker Sores

Local Medications

Other than the tetracycline "gargles" mentioned on page 132, there is no one, good, reliable, over-the-counter preparation that works for everybody. However, if you can't get to your physician or dentist, you can try the following preparation:

Proxigel (Reed & Carnrick)
Directions: Massage onto the affected areas 2 or 3 times daily.

Home Remedy

Or you can try treating your canker sores with tea bags at home. The tannic acid in tea, for some unexplained reason, helps to heal the sores.

Directions: Immerse a tea bag in water, remove it, and squeeze out most of the water. Then apply the tea bag directly to the canker sore. You may be pleasantly surprised at the result.

Rectal Itch

One bliss for which
There is no match
Is when you itch
To up and scratch.

Ogden Nash's little ditty doesn't include the socially unmentionable, tantalizing, embarrassing itch that torments the anal area, often incorrectly referred to as the rectal area. Known technically as pruritus ani (itching of the anal region), this stubborn condition has been known to cause sleepless nights, loss of work time, and severe emotional distress.

The single, most common cause of anal itch appears to be poor anal hygiene. In most parts of Europe and in many Eastern countries this ailment is almost non-existent. There people do not use toilet tissue—they *wash* the area. (The bidet is a much more distinctive sign of civilization than we Americans would like to think!) Other causative factors include the following:

- Hemorrhoids (piles) and other rectal disease, such as fissures, fistulas, or discharge after rectal surgery.
- Chronic diarrhea.
- Fungous and yeast infections in the area—often following long-term antibiotic therapy for other conditions.
- Pinworms and other parasitic infections, such as lice and mites (scabies).

- Psoriasis, seborrheic dermatitis, and eczema.
- Warts in the region.
- Diabetes.
- Diet. Coffee, spicy foods, chocolate, raw fruits and vegetables, alcoholic beverages, and other foods have sometimes been incriminated.
- Tight restrictive clothing—particularly the non-cotton varieties.
- Contact and irritative substances, such as topical anesthetic ointments and suppositories used for piles; colored, perfumed, and coarse toilet tissue; soaps (particularly the colored and scented varieties); anti-perspirants and deodorants; various hygiene sprays; bath salts; and—believe it or not—even nail polish has been implicated.
- Psychogenic causes. The itching occurs twice as often in men in their 40s and 50s than in women of the same age. This is thought to be due to certain stress situations (monetary for the most part) that develop in middle-aged men.

And then there are those cases where no cause has been determined—where careful study has failed to reveal any precipitating factor. This is by far the largest group and, unfortunately, the most resistant to treatment.

What can we do about pruritus ani? For prolonged, continuous, intolerable anal itching, see your physician. The following are some specific things you might do for at least temporary relief:

- Never use dry toilet paper. Instead, use cotton that has been soaked in warm water or an anal cleanser such as Balneol. And never wipe or rub! Blotting or patting are sufficient.
- Never use soap.
- Avoid irritants and contactants, such as bath salts, deodorants, sprays, perfumes, and colognes. Those perfumed fabric softeners used in clothes dryers should also be eliminated.
- Avoid tight, restrictive underclothing, pajamas, and pants. Wear only the loose, cotton varieties.

- For those who suspect a dietary cause, eliminate spicy foods, chocolate, coffee, alcohol, and raw fruits and vegetables.
- Discontinue all commercial, over-the-counter remedies in the form of salves and suppositories, particularly those containing benzocaine and other -caine derivatives. These may only aggravate the malady.
- If you suspect that emotional stress and tension are the cause, simmer down, stay cool, and relax.

For a severe, acute itching problem your physician will undoubtedly prescribe sitz baths in lukewarm water, a special prescription cream or ointment, and perhaps an anti-itch pill to break the itch-scratch reflex.

Treating Rectal Itch

For symptomatic relief of anal itching, first follow the rules on pages 135-136.

Cleanser

For anal cleansing, never use soap or toilet paper. Use the following instead:

Balneol (Geigy)

Local Medications

For added relief, use one of the following, compounded by your pharmacist:

Menthol	**0.1%**
Phenol	**¼%**
Cold Cream	**to make 2 oz.**

Directions: Apply every 4 hours and after each bowel movement.

Menthol	**0.1%**
Phenol	**¼%**
Burow's Solution	**10 cc**
Aquaphor	**20 gm**
Paste of Zinc Oxide	**to make 2 oz.**

Directions: Same as above.

Or use either of these over-the-counter preparations:

Rhulicort Cream (Lederle)
Vioform Cream 3% (Ciba)
Directions: Same as above.

For persistent, intractable itching, see your physician.

Lichen Planus

Lichen planus is a relatively common, harmless, itchy rash which involves the skin and mucous membranes. It occurs more commonly in the middle years, but any age group is susceptible.

It is characterized by reddish or violet-colored, shiny, flat-topped, diamond-shaped "bumps," called papules. This rash is usually symmetrical in appearance and most often involves the inner surfaces of the wrists and forearms, the ankles, and the lower portion of the back. In the rarer forms of the disease, blisters or thickened warty areas may appear.

No area of the skin surface, however, is immune from this condition. In the mouth, it can appear as a whitish or bluish-white, lacy-like pattern on the inner surface of the cheeks, or whitish patches over the sides of the tongue.

In addition, one out of 10 people with lichen planus has some type of nail changes, such as grooves, lines, distortion, or shedding of the nails.

The most characteristic symptom of lichen planus is itching. If there are only a few patches of lichen planus, the itching is usually mild. In the generalized form of the disease, however, the itching may be intense, causing loss of sleep, exhaustion, and despair.

The cause of lichen planus is unknown. It may be that lichen planus is not a disease at all—rather a symptom resulting from irritation, inflammation, or infection somewhere in the body.

Lichen planus rashes can occur in people taking certain drugs: high-blood pressure pills, antibiotics, as well as certain medications used to treat tuberculosis, malaria, and arthritis. The condition can also develop after exposure to a type of color film developer. Many cases of resistant lichen planus occur in association with long-standing, untreated ringworm infections of the feet (athlete's foot). Since the onset of lichen planus often coincides with some major emotional upset, it is often thought to be triggered by prolonged worry, anxiety, fatigue, shock, or other stressful situations.

Lichen planus can last for years, but, as a rule, the greater the involvement, the shorter the course. Generalized and extensive eruptions last anywhere from two months to two years. Localized eruptions, on the other hand, tend to remain considerably longer. And, unfortunately, recurrences are common, so one is never really sure that the condition has disappeared permanently.

While fairly common, lichen planus is not a condition that is easily recognized and diagnosed by the person who is afflicted. Or by relatives, friends, or the friendly pharmacist. Only a physician can make an accurate diagnosis, and while there is no specific therapy for lichen planus, your doctor will know how best to treat the rash and the itching that accompanies it.

Available treatments include various cortisone-type creams applied locally, certain antihistamine-tranquilizers taken orally, and cortisone-like injections into the patches of lichen planus. None of these, however, has shown more than limited success.

If you have a rash that has been diagnosed by your physician as lichen planus, be content to know that it is not contagious, infectious, serious, or malignant. Get as much rest as possible and avoid worry, tension, and fatigue. Maintain your general health and correct any hidden, internal infection you may have, such as abscessed teeth or infected gums.

Treating Lichen Planus

As discussed earlier, itching is probably the most obvious symptom of lichen planus. It is also one of the most difficult symptoms to contain.

Cream & Ointment

The localized patches of lichen planus are best managed with creams, ointments, and gels. The following preparations may provide some symptomatic relief:

Rhulicort Cream (Lederle)

Directions: Rub in gently 3 or 4 times daily to itchy areas.

Or have your pharmacist concoct the following:

Menthol	**¼%**
Phenol	**1%**
Cold Cream	**to make 4 oz.**

Directions: Rub in gently every 3 or 4 hours.

Baths, Lotions, & Liniments

Soothing baths, lotions, and liniments are more suitable for the extensive or widespread variety of lichen planus:

Balnetar (Westwood)

Directions: 2 to 4 capfuls to a tub of warm water.

Schamberg's Lotion (C & M Pharmacal)

Directions: Apply every 3 or 4 hours for the itching.

You can also have the pharmacist make up the following:

Menthol	**¼%**
Phenol	**½%**
Calamine Liniment (USP)	**to make 8 oz.**

Directions: Apply every 3 or 4 hours for the itching.

Oral Medications

For intense itching, take one of the following:

Chlor-Trimeton Tablets 4 mg (Schering)
Directions: One tablet every 4 hours for itching.

Dimetane Tablets 4 mg (Robins)
Directions: One tablet every 4 hours for itching.

For persistent, intractable itching, and when none of the above medications offers any relief, see your physician.

Vitiligo

Vitiligo is a mysterious malady characterized by a gradual loss of pigment, or skin color. It affects about one out of every hundred people and is more common among younger individuals.

No one knows what triggers this strange condition, but we do know that it results from a decrease or loss of the normal cells (melanocytes) which are responsible for the production of pigment (melanin) in the skin. This decrease generally shows up as white, sharply-bordered patches of different shapes and sizes on otherwise normal skin.

Vitiligo can occur on any portion of the skin surface, but more commonly involves the exposed parts, namely the face, neck, and backs of the hands. In severe cases the loss of pigment can extend over the entire body. The hairs in these depigmented patches also turn white, but if and when the pigment returns, it returns first in and around these hairs.

The pattern of vitiligo is unclear, although the condition appears to run in families. Most of the people afflicted are in good health. Occasionally, however, vitiligo occurs in association with such conditions as pernicious anemia, thyroid disease, diabetes, and disorders of the adrenal glands.

This pigmentary failure can occur in all races, but the cosmetic—as well as the psychological—implications are considerably greater for those with darker skins. In India, for example, vitiligo is considered by the populace to be a sure sign of leprosy. Nehru, realizing the myths and superstitions surrounding this perfectly benign condition, often remarked that a treatment for vitiligo was as important for his people as the treatment for leprosy and tuberculosis.

Vitiligo is usually a progressive and relentless disease, and rarely do people with the condition regain their color spontaneously. There may be a long period of time where the depigmented patches remain about the same. Very often, however, an emotional upset, infection, or illness may start the process again with the old spots getting larger and new spots developing.

Unfortunately, there is no reliable method of regaining lost pigment at the present time. Current therapy consists of taking a special pill and exposing the affected skin to sunlight or long-wave ultraviolet radiation. This form of therapy—commonly called the PUVA treatment—is similar to the way dermatologists treat extensive psoriasis. But even this procedure may have to be carried out for a number of months or years before any noticeable repigmentation occurs.

The prognosis for vitiligo is discouraging at best. Whatever the treatment only about one in five patients responds at all, and relapses are the rule. In some cases, particularly when the involved loss of pigment is in small patches, certain types of make-up (such as Covermark) and "stains" can help cover up the patches of vitiligo.

Treating Vitiligo

Dyes & Stains

The only methods of masking depigmented areas are with dyes, stains and cover-ups. I recommend the following:

Dy-O-Derm (Owen)
Vitadye (Elder)

These preparations contain the "staining" agent dihydroxyacetone. Directions for their use come with each bottle.

Cover-up

The following is a good, tinted, opaque make-up, in various shades that can effectively mask the areas of vitiligo:

Covermark (Lydia O'Leary)

Frostbite

Frostbite describes the sharp, painful sensations of freezing and thawing of the skin. It is a severe cold injury that, in many ways, resembles a thermal burn. Press an ice cube on your cheek for a few seconds. Burns, doesn't it? If you were to leave it there for a few minutes, a painful blister would develop.

Whether or not exposure to cold will result in frostbite depends on many factors. The degree of severity of frostbite is determined mainly by the temperature, the wind chill factor, the duration of exposure, and the adequacy of proper protective clothing. People's tolerance to cold varies as well. There are some factors that reduce one's tolerance, such as circulatory disease, poor general health, poor nutrition, fatigue, injury to a part of the body, immobility of an extremity, and contact with metals.

The areas of the body most vulnerable to the effects of frostbite are the tip of the nose, the rims and lobes of the ears, and the tips of the fingers and toes.

How do you recognize frostbite?

In its mildest form, known as frost nip, the skin suddenly turns pale due to the constriction of blood vessels. This is the body's method of conserving heat by diverting the blood to the vital organs. This skin pallor is accompanied by tingling. Burning and pain follow, and the skin becomes whitish or slightly yellow.

If the freezing continues, it affects the deeper tissues. The pain disappears, and there is a loss of sensation (numbness) in the areas affected. (Disappearance of pain is a warning sign of imminent danger!) The affected skin then becomes waxy white. If exposure to cold has been severe and of long duration, injury to deeper tissues, such as muscle, tendons, nerves, and bones, may follow. A recent study has shown that children who suffer severe cases of frostbitten fingers often end up with small hands as adults.

If you develop frostbite, see your physician at once. *Do not* treat it with ice, ice-water, or snow, as this results in the greatest amount of tissue death.

The best method to restore the normal temperature of the skin is by rapid rewarming of the frostbitten part. This treatment may produce more pain, more redness and swelling, and bigger blisters than gradual rewarming, but it promotes faster healing, reduces tissue loss, and prevents complications, such as infection, ulceration, gangrene, and even loss of a limb.

The recommended procedure is to immerse the affected part in a water bath at a temperature of 104° to 110° F (40° to 44° C), not higher, since it is possible to produce a burn in skin which lacks sensation.

Whirlpool baths are even better, but the use of local, dry heat is dangerous.

During the thawing process, blisters will develop which may persist for weeks while the newly formed skin may be tender for months.

Do not move any skin which is frozen; movement will result in severe damage. Also, don't smoke or drink alcohol.

To protect against frostbite, dress normally and protect those parts that are most susceptible to cold. When the temperature falls and the wind is howling, causing the chill factor to dip to arctic levels, protect those delicate sensitive areas: the fingertips with warm gloves or mittens; the ears with muffs or flaps; the nose with a ski mask; and the rest of the body with thermal underwear, long-johns, turtle neck sweaters, scarves, and fur-lined coats. Keep up your general health and avoid fatigue.

Treating Frostbite

Baths

The recommended procedure for frostbite is to immerse the affected part in a water bath at a temperature of 104° to 110° F (40° to 44° C).

Compresses

For the blisters which may develop during the thawing process, apply wet compresses for 15 to 20 minutes every 2 or 3 hours with any of the following antiseptic solutions to help dry them up:

AluWets Wet Dressing Crystals (Stiefel)
Directions: Dissolve contents of one packet in 12 ounces of warm water (again, the temperature should be 104° to 110° F) and apply as open dressings.

Bluboro Powder (Herbert)
Directions: Dissolve contents of one packet in a pint (16 ounces) of warm water and apply as above.

Domeboro Powder Packets (Dome)
Directions: Dissolve contents of one packet in a pint (16 ounces) of warm water and apply as above.

Lupus Erythematosus

Lupus erythematosus is one of those curious diseases that can masquerade as any of a dozen other medical maladies. Its variety of symptoms include fever, chills, headache, weakness, fatigue, hair loss, joint pains, chest pains, epileptic seizures, personality changes, and skin rashes. Any or all of these symptoms may usher in this strange complex that we commonly call LE.

What exactly is LE? It is a chronic inflammation of connective tissue—the so-called body "glue"—which binds our cells together. As such, it is considered a connective tissue, or collagen, disease and is often classified in the rheumatic group of diseases along with rheumatoid arthritis and rheumatic fever. Every portion of our body—all our organs, our muscles, blood, joints, skin—has this connective tissue, and thus, may be affected by LE.

No one really knows what causes LE. This puzzling condition is thought to be due to an "autoimmune process"—a technical way of saying that the body, due to some type of unexplained allergy, produces certain antibodies which attack its own tissues. A most difficult concept to comprehend.

It is important to know that there are two types of LE. One is the benign or "friendly" type which appears in localized patches on the skin. This is the so-called "discoid" variety of LE, which is commonly observed as red, scaly blotches symmetrically distributed over the sun-exposed areas of the body, notably the cheeks, nose, ears, scalp, the backs of the hands, and occasionally the "V" of the neck. If it affects the hairy regions of the beard or scalp, it usually results in permanent hair loss.

These lesions progress over a period of months or years, becoming larger and forming disc-shaped (hence, discoid) plaques. They slowly lose their reddish color, turn porcelain-white, and become depressed. This depression—essentially a scar—is the end result of a typical "discoid" lesion.

Triggered by some external factor, such as sunlight or injury, discoid LE affects all races, is more common in young adults, and occurs twice as often in women as in men. If you have discoid LE, it's important that you see your physician. While the condition itself is relatively harmless and poses little threat to your general health, these "discs" may be harbingers of some underlying condition that can flare up into systemic lupus erythematosus (SLE).

SLE is a serious variety of LE that can affect and damage any or all of the bodily organs or systems: kidneys, liver, heart, lungs, bone marrow, and joints. Fortunately, only about one in ten patients with discoid LE ever progresses to the systemic or internal type of the disease.

One of the triggering mechanisms that may convert the "friendly" condition into the more serious, "unfriendly" variety is sun exposure. Other factors are stress, injury, fatigue, overwork, and various medications, such as those used for high blood pressure, heart disease, and epilepsy; certain antibiotics and birth control pills; and various types of tranquilizers.

Your doctor may prescribe certain cortisone-type creams and ointments to reduce the redness and relieve the inflammation in the affected patches. While internal remedies are rarely needed for the discoid variety of LE, progressive, widespread, or disfiguring lesions may require drugs called antimalarials to prevent further spread.

Treating LE

Sunblocks & Sunscreens

The treatment for LE is up to your physician. However, to prevent aggravating the condition, always use a sun-protective agent before exposure to the sun's rays. Any of the following will do:

PreSun 15 (Westwood)
Total Eclipse (Herbert)
Super Shade (Plough)
Solbar Plus 15 (Persōn & Covey)
Directions for the above are on the labels of each container or tube.

Cream

For itching associated with LE patches, try the following:

Rhulicort Cream (Lederle)
Directions: Apply 3 times daily.

Diaper Rash & Prickly Heat

Two common skin conditions associated with infants and children are diaper rash and prickly heat. While neither condition is serious or dangerous, when left untreated either can lead to widespread infection by bacteria or fungi necessitating vigorous and prolonged treatment.

Fortunately, both conditions are easily preventable.

Diaper Rash

Diaper rash, the bane of young mothers, the frustration of young fathers, and often the challenge of seasoned pediatricians, is one of the most common skin disorders. Frequently beginning between the ages of 2 and 4 months, this itchy, nasty-looking rash can persist for months or until your child outgrows diapers.

Also known as napkin or diaper dermatitis, diaper rash is any eruption on an infant's buttocks, genital and anal areas, lower abdomen, and upper thighs that develops during the diaper-wearing period. While the problem is usually minor, the rash frequently recurs. And, when ignored, it can cause complications in the form of impetigo and fungous infections.

In its earliest and simplest form, diaper rash is characterized by redness or chafing of the skin covered by the diaper. If left untreated, small pimples, called papules, and water blisters, or vesicles, develop. These can lead to oozing, sogginess in the folds of the skin and, in severe cases, open sores. The rash is usually accompanied by the sharp, pungent odor of ammonia.

The most common villain which promotes this contact is the infant's rubber or plastic pants which constrict and prevent the skin from "breathing." The irritation may be further aggravated by the rough edges of such pants as well as by tightly-pinned diapers.

Be especially careful if the infant has diarrhea. Frequent loose stools with their noxious intestinal enzymes further irritate the delicate diaper area, especially when these stools have not been completely removed by cleaning. Other causes of irritation include harsh soaps for cleaning the skin; strong detergents, antiseptic rinses, and perfumed fabric softeners for diapers; as well as certain baby oils, salves, ointments, and other chemical irritants.

High heat and humidity also contribute to diaper rash, since they can cause the skin and skin folds to become waterlogged. This, in turn, creates an inflammatory reaction around the sweat pores which prevents the normal flow of secretions. The inflammation lowers the resistance of the skin to infection. The normal, usually "friendly" germs, such as bacteria and fungi, then begin to thrive in the trapped secretions and become "unfriendly."

Dismal as this situation seems, there are some positive steps you can take to prevent and treat diaper rash. Here are some suggestions for prevention:

- Change diapers as soon as they have been soiled *and* at regular intervals. Be on the alert and learn to anticipate.
- Use plastic and rubber pants only sparingly and for short periods of time, such as for party occasions. Never use them at night.
- Following each diaper change, clean the diaper area thoroughly but gently with a mild soap, such as Dove, to remove all bacterial and fecal contamination. Pay careful attention to the skin folds. These folds should be washed and then rinsed thoroughly to ensure that all soapy solution is completely removed.
- Thoroughly dry the skin and skin folds.

- Use a medicated cornstarch-based powder 2 or 3 times daily to keep the affected areas dry. Do *not* use talcum powder. Recent research suggests that this common product, which has been dusted on babies' bottoms for over 80 years, causes tumors—called granulomas—when dusted on broken or abraded skin. (The government of Puerto Rico recently banned talc, used in manufacturing rice, due to its suspected link to stomach cancer.)
- Wash diapers in mild soap or detergent. Make sure they are thoroughly rinsed.
- Don't use fabric softeners, particularly those perfumed pads used in drying machines.
- Dress the child in clothing that is porous enough to allow good air circulation.
- Keep air in the child's room cool and dry.
- Encourage early training in regular toilet habits.

If your child is already suffering from a bout of diaper rash, the following steps can help clear up and prevent further irritation, inflammation, and infection:

- Discontinue all previous medication.
- Discontinue plastic and rubber pants.
- Do not use soap when the area is inflamed.
- Use compresses, wet dressings, or 10- to 15-minute baths using Burow's Solution (2 Domeboro packets dissolved in one quart of warm water) every 3 or 4 hours to soothe and cool the inflamed areas.
- Permit the affected areas to "breathe." Air is a marvelous healing agent. I strongly recommend that children with diaper rash be permitted to lie about and run around naked for several hours a day!

During the acute stage of diaper rash, I recommend discontinuing *all* diapers during the day. And use a double layer of soft, cotton diapers, very loosely pinned, at night. Never use plastic or rubber pants at any time. When the inflammation, oozing, and sogginess have begun to clear and dry up, use a soothing preparation, such as Methakote Diaper Rash Cream, at night. Finally, when the affected areas have sufficiently healed and the child is more comfortable and less irritable, you may use soft cotton diapers again.

Be especially careful and conscientious, change the sheets as often as necessary, cleanse the soiled areas gently but thoroughly, and re-apply the Methakote Diaper Rash Cream after each soiling.

Prickly Heat

Prickly heat is a common disorder of the sweat apparatus. It occurs when the free flow of sweat to the surface of the skin is obstructed.

Sweat is produced by more than 2 million sweat glands in the skin. Under normal conditions, it flows out smoothly and continuously to the skin surface by means of tiny sweat ducts. If the sweat is heavy and prolonged, it can block the ducts and become trapped. This trapped sweat, unable to reach the skin surface, breaks through the walls of the ducts. The result is an inflammation of the skin known as prickly heat, or heat rash.

Prickly heat takes the form of numerous, tiny, reddish pimples and water blisters scattered in the creases of the neck, under the chin, and on the chest, back, abdomen, and buttocks. It appears suddenly and can cause restlessness, irritability, and burning and prickling sensations.

Prickly heat can result from any condition that promotes profuse and prolonged sweating and inadequate evaporation of the sweat. The culprit can be an excessively hot and humid climate or a fever. It is aggravated by obesity and tight-fitting garments. It usually clears up on its own fairly quickly, and only rarely do complications, in the form of secondary bacterial and fungal infections, occur. While it lasts, however, it can be very distressing, particularly for children.

Fortunately, there are some simple and effective methods to prevent and treat prickly heat. The primary consideration is to keep the *skin* cool and dry. This is accomplished by keeping the *air* cool and dry. Some helpful hints include the following:

- Use an air-conditioner or fan to reduce the temperature and humidity.
- Provide adequate room ventilation to help sweat evaporate.
- Wear loose-fitting, lightweight cotton clothing and limit physical activity in hot, humid weather.

If prickly heat has already taken hold, try the following treatment:

- Apply soothing and drying lotions, such as calamine lotion.
- Use a 100% talc-free cornstarch-based dusting powder. (Do *not* use talcum powder.)
- If possible, allow the afflicted person to lie about the house naked.
- Wash with a soap-substitute, such as Lowila Cake, and never use greases or ointments, which will further clog the sweat ducts.
- During the acute phase of prickly heat, take lukewarm baths, preferably with starch or Aveeno Oatmeal.

Of course, the main answer to prickly heat is to stay cool!

Treating Diaper Rash

Wet Dressings

For the weeping and oozing of acute diaper rash, use soothing wet dressings of the following to help relieve the inflammation and make the child more comfortable:

Domeboro Powder Packets (Dome)

Directions: Dissolve contents of one packet in 1 pint (16 oz.) of warm water and apply as open wet dressings for 15 to 20 minutes every 2 to 3 hours. (See page 208 for directions for applying wet dressings.)

Cream

After the acute inflammation has subsided with the wet dressings, apply the following cream:

Methakote Diaper Rash Cream (Syntex)

Directions: Apply at night to the affected areas.

Treating Prickly Heat

Bath

Aveeno Colloidal Oatmeal (Cooper)

Directions: See directions on the label.

Soap Substitutes

Lowila Cake (Westwood)

Aveenobar (Cooper)

Powder

Diaparene Baby Powder (Glenbrook)

Tinea Versicolor

Tinea versicolor is a friendly, minor fungous infection of the skin. *Friendly* means that it is relatively harmless. *Minor* means that it is only mildly contagious (through direct contact and clothing) and—for the most part—is easy to cure. However, it can be itchy and, when widespread, may be embarrassing cosmetically.

Like most fungous infections, tinea versicolor thrives in hot, humid environments. And, while some people appear to be more susceptible to this condition than others, it is generally more common among adolescents and young adults.

The name tinea versicolor means "superficial fungous infection characterized by a change of color." Under the microscope, the fungus looks like a dish of spaghetti and meatballs—small spherical spores and rod-like filaments. (It is thus referred to by dermatologists as the "spaghetti-and-meatball" fungus.)

To the eye, tinea versicolor appears as fine, round, scaly patches that usually are tan or fawn-colored. These patches are most common over the chest, back, and shoulders. Acting as a sunscreen, they block out the sun's rays. In white people, this results in depigmented areas of the skin that are lighter than the surrounding, tanned skin in summer and darker than the surrounding, untanned skin in winter. In black people, these depigmented patches can be various colors, such as tan, brown, gray, yellow, or pink.

To diagnose tinea versicolor, a physician gently scrapes a patch to remove a grayish scale. This scale is the actual fungous colony which lives only in the outer, dead layers of the skin. If this scale shows the typical spaghetti-and-meatball pattern under the microscope, the diagnosis is confirmed.

Fortunately, tinea versicolor is easy to treat and leaves no scars. However, since the condition has a tendency to recur, particularly in hot, humid weather, treatment may have to continue over a long period of time. And, if left untreated, the condition may persist indefinitely.

Treatment usually consists of washing the affected areas with a prescription-type shampoo containing selenium sulfide. Over-the-counter soaps and shampoos containing sulfur and salicylic acid, such as Fostex Medicated Cleansing Bar or Fostex Medicated Cleansing Cream, also can do a pretty good job. Washing the affected areas for a full five minutes once daily for a period of two weeks will usually eliminate most of the active fungus. Monthly washings should prevent the condition from recurring. In addition, I recommend thoroughly shampooing the scalp with Fostex Medicated Cleansing Cream at least once weekly, since the fungus often sets up housekeeping in the back of the scalp. Other shampoos can be used in between.

Even after the fungus has been destroyed, the patches may require repeated sun exposure to change back to their normal color. This may take months, so be patient!

Treating Tinea Versicolor

Fostex Medicated Cleansing Bar or **Fostex Medicated Cleansing Cream** (Westwood)

Directions: Wash affected areas thoroughly for five minutes daily for a period of two weeks. Repeat these washings monthly for a year or longer.

Shampoo scalp at least once weekly with Fostex Medicated Cleansing Cream.

7 Cosmetic Problems

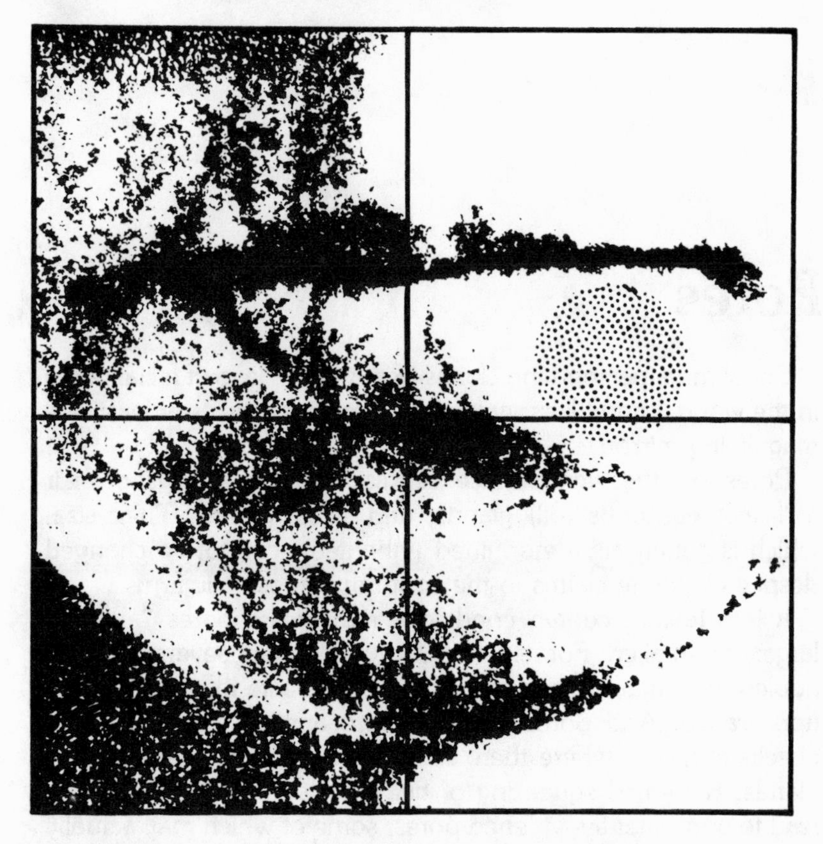

There are many conditions of the skin that are not really diseases in the sense that they are contagious, infectious, malignant, or serious. There is no infection, no inflammation, nothing to worry about medically. These, to all intents and purposes, are essentially cosmetic problems.

Some are normal conditions which occur as we "mature"; some are abnormal formations (scars, stretch marks, and keloids), as a result of some type of injury to the skin.

These benign, or "friendly," conditions and problems are discussed in the following sections.

Pores

Show me a person who claims to have the "largest facial pores in the world," and I'll show you someone who owns at least one magnifying mirror!

Pores on the skin surface represent the openings of hair follicles, sebaceous (oil) glands, and sweat glands. Their size, which is genetically determined (inherited), cannot be changed despite elaborate claims to the contrary by cosmetic firms.

It is true that certain conditions may make pores "appear" larger or smaller. For example, oily skin and severe acne in adolescence may distend the oil ducts to create the "large pore" appearance. And pores may be more apparent on the nose, cheeks and chin where there is the greatest concentration of oil glands. Repeated squeezing of blackheads and "zits" may also lead to permanently-widened pores, some of which may actually be tiny, pitted scars.

Other factors can temporarily make your pores look smaller. For instance, note what happens to your pores when you get a sunburn. They become considerably smaller, due to the inflammation and swelling around the pores. Of course, once the inflammation has subsided, the pores return to their original appearance. Pinching or gently slapping the skin of the cheeks to make them pink has a similar, temporary pore-shrinking effect.

There is *no* scientific evidence to support the fact that pores can be made to open and close, as many advertisements would lead us to believe. However, certain astringents containing alcohol and acetone, as well as various facial masks, remove excess oil from the skin surface. This makes the skin feel cool and tight, giving the impression that these enlarged pores are, indeed, shrinking. A possible explanation of this mechanism is that the astringent or mask acts as an irritant on the skin surface. This irritation causes a swelling of the skin surrounding the pore, thus making the opening appear smaller and shrunken. Any shrinkage, however, is so minuscule and so transitory that the time, effort, and cost involved for achieving this short-lived effect are usually not worth the outcome.

Much as I hate to shatter any preconceived notions and grandmothers' tales, hot baths, hot showers, and hot packs followed by cold baths, cold showers, and cold packs do absolutely nothing to the size of the pores. The only effect this "hot-cold" theory has is to make one feel that something—a contraction, a tightening, a shriveling, whatever—is actually going on in these pores. And this salutary psychological effect is not to be ridiculed. If it makes you feel good—do it! It cannot do any harm.

For those of you out there who think your facial pores are the largest, the ugliest, and the most noticeable, do the following:

- Cleanse your skin thoroughly with soap and water to prevent oils from accumulating, clogging up, and distending the pores.
- Use any good, commercial astringent or face mask that makes you and your skin feel good.
- Use only water-based and oil-free cosmetics.
- And throw away your magnifying mirrors...

Wrinkles

Wrinkles—those bitter reminders of the aging process—are a natural phenomenon that occurs in all of us.

As we get on in years, the skin, for a number of reasons, begins to lose its elasticity, its flexibility, and its resiliency. It becomes thinner, fine lines develop, and then—horror of horrors—wrinkles.

What really happens to our skin as we grow older? The sweat glands and oil glands, which for many years have provided moisture and lubrication to the skin, get tired, work less, and diminish in size and number. The greater portion of the oils which have made the skin smooth and supple, as well as the fluid from the sweat glands which has kept the cells plumped up and rounded, have for the most part disappeared, leaving the surface dry and cracked.

The fibers that support the skin begin to lose their strength and elasticity. Remember the old elevated trains? Just imagine that the pillars—the structures supporting the tracks—suddenly begin to bend, break, or crumble. What happens to the train and the tracks? All fall down...That's basically what happens to the skin. The supporting collagen and elastic fibers deteriorate, and the skin begins to sag over the broken and crumbled understructure.

There is also a decrease in the amount of beneficial hormones delivered to the skin cells. As a result, the fat pads in the skin begin to shrink and certain fibers, which attach the skin to the muscles, relax and become weak, causing sagging and wrinkles.

How much you wrinkle and at what age are influenced by other factors as well:

- Excessive washing and scrubbing, particularly with harsh soaps and very hot water, contribute to the breakage of the elastic fibers and tend to dissolve the essential oils that help nourish the skin.
- Exaggerated facial expressions, such as excessive laughing and frowning, and rough massages and facial exercises also weaken the elastic fibers and lead to premature wrinkling: horizontal lines of the forehead, "crow's feet" about the eyes, "laugh lines," and others.
- Sudden weight loss, due to diet or disease, also contributes to lines and wrinkles. After having been stretched out of shape for many years, the skin is unable to retract and so begins to hang in folds. This is similar to what happens to a person's clothes after he or she loses a lot of weight. They become loose, baggy, and begin to sag in folds. As our bones and fat and muscles shrink, the skin around them becomes loose and baggy.
- Hereditary factors also play a role in wrinkles. People with thin skin—the Irish and Scottish, for example—age more rapidly than "thick-skinned" individuals.
- Excessive smoking is thought to be a contributory factor in the formation of wrinkles. Did you ever notice how smokers screw up their faces to prevent smoke from getting in their eyes? This, coupled with a decrease in the circulation of blood to the facial skin, is said to cause premature lines and wrinkles.
- Exposure to the elements (heat, cold, wind, and particularly sunlight) hasten and aggravate the natural aging process. You'll notice that the skin of the buttocks shows none of the degenerative and aging changes that are observed on the skin exposed to the sun—the face, neck, hands, and forearms. The covered portions of your body are young; your sun-exposed portions are old.

Aging and wrinkling vary from person to person, so there is no hard and fast rule to pinpoint the exact decade when a person will begin experiencing these hallmarks of decline. As a rule, however, in the 40s and 50s, there is a progressive shrinking of body substance—bone, fat, muscle, and fluid—but *not* of skin. This loss of tissue volume, coupled with the decrease of the elasticity of the skin, leads to sagging.

It occurs first where the skin is thinnest: the eyelids, neck, and jaw lines. Jowls develop, the neck becomes creased, lines begin to radiate from the mouth, and "crow's feet" and "bags" develop about the eyes. All this is due to the fact that there is too much facial skin to cover the reduced volume of underlying tissue.

Can we do anything about wrinkles? Yes, but there are no types of creams, potions, facial masks, exercises, or massages that can flatten out or permanently erase lines and wrinkles.

Mink oil, turtle oil, placenta extract and other expensive rejuvenating creams, "wrinkle creams," and facial masks do nothing more than offer temporary relief from dryness by lubricating and softening the roughened, weather-beaten skin. Likewise, those facial saunas and the "electric needle" treatments have no lasting effect on dryness, lines, or wrinkles.

Masks, saunas, and the like can have some psychological benefits, but let's not fool ourselves. Their permanent effect on the skin is nil. However, they probably won't harm you either—so if it makes you feel good, do it!

The only procedures that will improve lines and wrinkles are forms of cosmetic surgery. "Face-lifts'" by plastic surgeons (and some dermatologists) can smooth the skin of the cheeks and forehead, remove the "bags" about the eyes, and eliminate the loose, flabby skin of the neck.

There are some things you can do while you're young to forestall the wrinkling process:

- Avoid the sun! I cannot stress this enough. In otherwise healthy individuals, sun exposure is the prime cause not only of wrinkles, aging skin, and other degenerative changes, but of skin cancers. If you do want to soak up all that ultraviolet radiation, use a protective sunscreen. This will screen out some—

but not all—of those harmful, wrinkle-producing rays.

- Avoid extremes of heat and cold, and protect your face against the wind and rain and snow.
- Wash your face gently and avoid overly-hot water and harsh soaps.
- Do not lose and gain weight—off again, on again—like a yo-yo. The constant expansion and contraction of the skin will only tire out the elastic fibers.
- No facial exercises or isometrics. These, when overdone, can also cause a breakdown of the elastic fibers and collagen in the skin.
- And cut down on smoking.

If you already have wrinkles and if they are causing you great concern, your only other option (if you can afford it) is cosmetic surgery. The rewards can be great, but only you can decide whether you want to alter nature—or let it takes its course.

Scars

Almost everyone has a scar. From vaccinations, cuts and lacerations, burns, acne, boils, chicken pox, shingles, or surgical procedures or operations.

Scars are permanent. The hucksters who thrive on misrepresentation would have you believe that they have "proven" products that will flatten out or eliminate scars. Don't believe them! Massaging scars with various creams and potions containing such magical ingredients as turtle oil, placenta extract, collagen, or vitamin E is useless and expensive. Some scars can, however, be made less conspicuous by skin planing (dermabrasion) or by treatment with various acids. Such procedures are best done by a plastic surgeon or dermatologist trained in these areas.

Since the incidence of cancer in scars (particularly those due to burns) is higher than in normal skin, it is important to consult a physician if you notice any changes in an old scar.

The following sections discuss two special types of scars: stretch marks and keloids.

Stretch Marks

Stretch marks are very thin scars that commonly develop when the skin is distended, or stretched, for a long period of time. This strains the elastic fibers in the deeper layers of the skin to the point where they cannot regain their initial resiliency. As a result, the skin is unable to revert to its original condition.

The most common sites for stretch marks are the abdomen, hips, buttocks, thighs, and breasts. They are usually associated with puberty (when young girls and boys tend to fill out very rapidly), obesity, and pregnancy. However, they have also been linked to certain glandular disturbances; severe illnesses, such as scarlet fever or typhoid; and salves and lotions containing cortisone-like preparations, when used in body folds over long periods of time or applied under plastic film to treat certain skin diseases.

Stretch marks are initially reddish or purple. After many months, however, the color usually fades out and these shallow scars become white.

There are no measures in the form of lotions, creams or ointments that can modify or erase these scars. Plastic surgeons have recently recommended a rather complicated surgical procedure that involves excising a great deal of skin, tightening up the underlying muscles, and following all this up with dermabrasion (skin planing). Before you contemplate such a drastic measure, however, keep in mind that the only problem stretch marks cause is possibly a cosmetic one.

To prevent stretch marks, don't gain too much weight during pregnancy, avoid extreme tension on the skin, and never get fat.

Keloids

A keloid is an abnormal scar, a bizarre response to injury. Actually, it is an overgrowth of scar tissue. The scar tissue continues to form long after it is needed, building up extra tissue and resulting in a hard, smooth, and round lump.

We don't know what causes keloids. Neither can we predict when and in whom they will occur and to what size they may develop. For some reason, they are much more common in Orientals and blacks, who may develop keloids after slight or insignificant injuries.

While keloids are entirely harmless, they may create a cosmetic problem. In rare instances they may be somewhat incapacitating, for example, if they develop across joints. They are also highly resistant to treatment.

If the keloid is small and inconspicuous, let it be. For larger lesions and those that are cosmetically unacceptable, your physician can offer a variety of treatments—but no guarantees that they will work. These can include injections of a cortisone-like suspension directly into the keloid; surgical excision followed by the cortisone injections (surgical excision alone will only result in a recurrence of the keloid which may then become larger than the original lesion); X-ray treatment; and freezing the area with liquid nitrogen or dry ice. The type of treatment depends on the age, size, and location of the keloids. Older keloids are less responsive to treatment, and the larger the keloid, the more difficult it is to treat.

Cellulite

According to a recent best-seller on the subject, cellulite (pronounced cell-you-leet) is a "household word in Europe." It is used to describe the "lumps, bumps, and bulges" that do not disappear with simple diet and exercise. What it doesn't say is that cellulite will affect practically every female, regardless of age.

Cellulite is an invented disease. It is a "normal abnormality," a cosmetic blight that has tortured European women for many decades. The proponents of this non-disease, seeking new markets for their advertising and useless remedies, have begun to flood the American market with their "miracle" products and their fraudulent claims.

What is this phenomenon, and how does it manifest itself? If you are a woman, make this pinch test: With your palms about four inches apart, press and squeeze together the outer part of your upper thigh. If the skin ripples and looks like a mattress, it means you have cellulite. It also probably means that you are a woman!

In a recent scientific investigation of almost 1,000 women of various ages, this mattress phenomenon occurred in practically all of them. Cellulite is not found in men who have the normal amount of male hormones (androgens). However, this mattress phenomenon is found in men who have an androgen deficiency due to hormonal disease.

Cellulite is a sex-typical feature of women's skin and is *not* a sign of disease. The buttocks and thighs are the most common sites, but this condition can also occur over the lower part of the abdomen, the upper portions of the arms, and other locations. Contrary to reports in non-medical literature, cellulite is not painful, nor is it due to illness, miniskirts, or oral contraceptives.

What do hormones have to do with cellulite, and why do only women have it? The following is a simplified, non-technical explanation.

The skin of the average woman—who has little, if any, male hormones—is significantly thinner than that of a man. As women age, this thin skin becomes even thinner and looser. This lost skin is replaced by clusters of fat cells. It is these fatty clusters—high up in the skin—that are responsible for the mattress phenomenon and the feel of cellulite.

What can we do about cellulite and how can we prevent or minimize it? The paperback best-sellers, advertisements, and commercials would have us believe that diet, proper bowel function, breathing exercises, relaxation, yoga, massage, enzyme injections (popular in France) or the heralded "rice treatment" can eliminate this hallmark of womanhood. According to medical experts, however, there is only one way to prevent cellulite and that is to avoid becoming overweight.

If you are overweight, slow and progressive weight loss and exercising to improve muscle tone in the buttocks and thighs may help reduce cellulite. (Female athletes, incidentally, show little or no cellulite.)

It seems a pity, however, that what was once fashionable and "ideal," as depicted by such famous artists as Botticelli, Rubens and Goya, is no longer considered chic.

Sweat

All normal, healthy people sweat. Some more, some less. People also smell when they sweat. This, too, is normal.

Sweat is important in regulating our body temperature. Despite enormous changes in the temperature of our external environment—be it at the North Pole or at the Equator—our internal body temperature remains fairly constant.

When we are exposed to excessive heat, the sweat glands pour out their watery secretion (sweat) which then cools our body by evaporation. By virtue of this thermo-regulatory mechanism, humans have been able to adapt themselves to the hottest climates.

Sweat is composed of the secretion of two types of glands: the eccrine glands (over 2 million of them), which are widely distributed over the body, and the localized apocrine glands, which are restricted primarily to the armpits (axillae), the anogenital region, and the nipples. The growth of these apocrine glands is regulated by a hormone which begins to form about the time of puberty and decreases markedly in old age. This is why children below the age of twelve and elderly people do not suffer from "body odor."

Perspiration is not under voluntary control. We cannot decide when we want to perspire and we cannot tell ourselves to stop this mechanism. Emotional and environmental factors (heat) influence the degree of sweating, and it is believed that cigarette smoking may also be responsible for excessive perspiration.

Anti-perspirants are compounds which reduce the volume of perspiration. Deodorants are products used to mask, diminish, or prevent perspiration odor.

Anti-Perspirants

While it is not certain how anti-perspirants act, it is believed that they reduce perspiration by strictly mechanical means. Made up almost exclusively of aluminum salts, anti-perspirants are sold as pads, creams, sprays, lotions, powders, liquids, and roll-ons.

None of these products will completely stop the flow of perspiration. And since the secretion of sweat is an essential function of the skin for temperature regulation and water metabolism, it would not be desirable if they did. As for safely limiting control of perspiration, it should be noted that in order to be considered a true anti-perspirant, the product must reduce perspiration by at least 25%.

Roll-ons and creams usually give greater protection than aerosols, but the choice of one type over another is a matter of personal preference: ease of application, lack of messiness, the absence of burning or stinging, and which TV commercial appeals to you. In very severe cases of excessive perspiration, your physician can prescribe certain oral drugs. These, however, can have certain undesirable side effects which might preclude their continuous use.

Deodorants

Sweat itself is essentially odorless. The odor is due to the action of various bacteria on the milky secretion of the apocrine sweat glands. These bacteria are most active in moist and warm environments.

The popular topical preparations used to prevent these odors have included such antibacterial agents as hexachlorophene (recently banned by the Food and Drug Administration for over-the-counter use), neomycin, salicylanilides (found in certain deodorant soaps), and other bacteria-destroying chemicals. These compounds, unlike the perfumes, colognes, and toilet waters of a previous era which merely masked perspiration odor, work by reducing or eliminating the offending bacteria. They do not in any way affect the flow of perspiration. Deodorants may be purchased as powders, creams, sticks, pads, roll-ons, soaps, or sprays, and are effective for a few hours to several days. For those who are allergic to the popular, commercial deodorant preparations, there are so-called "hypoallergenic" products.

Deodorants which do not claim to check perspiration are classified as cosmetics. If the same preparation is labeled an "anti-perspirant," it becomes a drug, as it claims to change a bodily function.

The best methods of controlling body odor, however, are personal cleanliness (frequent bathing) and thorough cleaning and laundering of clothing which has collected not only the odors, but the germs which have produced these odors.

Is it difficult to get rid of perspiration odor? No sweat!

Dry Skin

Dry skin is a loose, unscientific term that generally refers to the rough, scaly, and flaky skin that is dry to the touch and less flexible, or "elastic," than normal skin. And lest anyone think otherwise, let me set the record straight: dry skin does *not* cause wrinkles.

Dryness of the skin usually develops as winter approaches. When the temperature drops and the relative humidity decreases, the upper layers of the skin lose a large amount of water, leading to dryness, scaling, and occasional itching.

This decrease in humidity is further aggravated by artificial heating, which, in addition to warming the air, dries it out. The air, in turn, draws moisture from objects in the vicinity—plants, furniture, and skin. (As the relative humidity drops we become aware of it by means of the familiar, slight, unexpected shocks that result from a build-up of static electricity.)

Dry skin tends to improve spontaneously during the summer months, and wherever there is high relative humidity.

Dry skin was originally thought to be entirely due to a deficiency in the oily film on the surface of the skin. We now know that it is due primarily to the loss of water from the outer layers of our skin and to the inability of moisture to move from the deeper layers to the surface. While the natural oils on the surface of the skin act to prevent the excess evaporation of water from the lower layers, these oils really have little to do with preventing skin dryness if there isn't enough moisture in the cells to begin with.

Dry skin is influenced by several factors. It is more common in the elderly where, despite adequate water content of the skin, there are diminished oily secretions. Overheated homes with markedly lowered humidity also play a role in promoting excessive dryness. The combination of strong, alkaline soaps, coupled with the fetish of many individuals for very hot, long, and frequent baths, is probably the greatest cause of dry skin.

Other contributing factors include excessive sun-bathing and overexposure to wind and cold; rough, woolen, and fuzzy clothing; linens which have been laundered in harsh detergents and inadequately rinsed; and nutritional deficiencies arising from some of the recent faddist diets.

Here are some general guidelines for avoiding dry skin:

- Increase the relative humidity in your home to at least 40% by properly adjusting the heating or air-conditioning systems. If this is not practicable, buy a good, commercial room humidifier.
- Do not bathe or shower in very hot water and avoid harsh alkaline soaps.
- Avoid excessive sun-bathing, cold temperatures, and strong winds.
- Do not wear heavy, woolen, fuzzy clothing.
- Maintain your general health and correct any nutritional deficiencies by means of a well-balanced diet and adequate water intake.

Specific methods of therapy include bland soaps, soothing bath oils, and various water-attracting creams and lotions which help retard the evaporation of moisture from the skin surface and leave the skin smooth, soft, and supple.

Treating Dry Skin

Products for dry skin include bath oils, emollient creams and lotions, and soaps.

Bath Oils

Since dry skin results from lack of water, an excellent way to replenish this loss is by bathing in water to which bath oils have been added. These oils are adsorbed onto the skin ("coat the body," so to speak). By doing this, they seal in the needed water that helps to plump up the skin cells to make the skin more soft and pliable. (A note of caution! All bath oils make the bathtub slippery. Be careful! They also make bathtubs difficult to clean.)

I suggest that you try any of the following bath oils:

Aveeno Oilated (Cooper)
Alpha Keri Therapeutic Bath Oil (Westwood)
nutraSpa Bath Oil (Owen)
Surfol Post-Immersion Bath Oil (Stiefel)
Lubath (Parke-Davis)

Directions: Follow the directions given on the container.

Emollients

The following emollient preparations act mainly to soften and lubricate:

Keri Lotion (Westwood)
Neutrogena Lotion (Neutrogena)
Nutraderm Lotion (Owen)
Mī-Skin Lotion (Michel)
Lubriderm Lotion (Parke-Davis)
Shepard's Cream Lotion (Dermik)
Wibi Dry Skin Lotion (Owen)
Nivea Creme Lotion (Beiersdorf)

Moisturizers

The following moisturizing preparations for excessively dry skin contain special ingredients to counteract dryness and itching and help make the skin more supple and resilient:

Carmol-10 Lotion (Syntex)
LactiCare Lotion (Stiefel)
Nutraplus Lotion (Owen)
Aquacare/HP Lotion (Herbert)
Purpose Dry Skin Cream (Johnson & Johnson)

Soaps

If you suffer from dry skin, avoid harsh alkaline soaps, as these tend to degrease the skin surface. The following are soaps and cleansers which contain substances that help restore those oils which have been lost in the dry skin process.

Alpha Keri Soap (Westwood)
Neutrogena Dry Skin Soap (Neutrogena)
Oilatum Soap (Stiefel)
Basis Soap (Beiersdorf)
Emulave (Cooper)

Cream

For especially dry skin, try the following cream:

Carmol-20 Cream (Syntex)
Directions: Follow the directions on the label.

8 Hair Care and Scalp Diseases

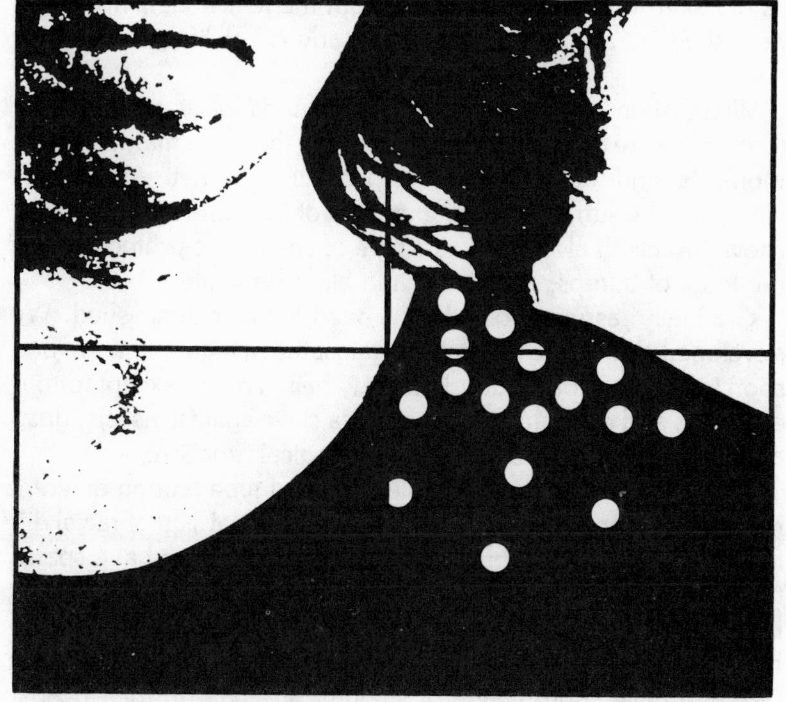

Hair—our crowning glory.

And yet, depending upon where it grows, how much, and upon whom, hair can be either a blessing or a curse.

We cut it, shave it, twirl it, comb it, and brush it in a fashion to make it appear longer and more abundant. Some of us tease, tint, dye, bleach, spray, iron, roll, and frost it. We straighten curly hair, and we curl straight hair. Blondes become brunettes, and vice versa.

We tear our hair. We split hairs. We let our hair down. We make our hair stand on end, and we get in someone else's hair.

What is this culturally, socially, and sexually significant ornamental appendage we refer to as hair? It is a non-living, protein fiber, a strong, elastic thread, arising from a long indentation—a follicle or "pore"—in the skin.

Hair is dead. Although it is as integral a component of the body as our skin, once it has emerged from the follicle, it is no longer nourished by a blood-supply or by any other life-giving bodily fluids.

What, then, is its purpose? Thousands of years ago our forebears were covered with hair in much the same manner as the monkeys and apes. It was a protective barrier against the elements: the sun, the wind, extremes of heat and cold, rain and snow, insects. It also acted as a type of cushion to protect against the force of bumps, abrasions, and blows in battle.

Gradually, as we evolved, our need for hair diminished. We developed clothing to protect us against the ravages of nature and soon lost most of our redundant body hair. Today, except for our eyebrows and eyelashes which act as a sieve against insects, dust, and other irritants, hair serves no biological function.

Hair varies in color, texture, length, and type among different races. It is second only to skin color as a physical sign of racial difference. Orientals, Eskimos, and American Indians have sparse facial and body hair and straight, coarse, dark hairs on their heads. Blacks have slightly more body hair and woolly or wiry hair on their scalps. Whites have more body hair than any other race and have curly, wavy, or straight, fine hair on their heads.

The amount and color of our hair are determined by the genes we inherit from our parents. In addition, we each generally have three types of hair: the long, soft, terminal hairs, such as those on the scalp, armpits, and pubic region; the short, stiff, coarse hairs of the eyelids, eyebrows, nose, and ears; and the soft, fine, downy fuzz (known as lanugo or vellus hairs) which covers the rest of the body, except the palms and soles, the lips, the nipples, and certain parts of the genitals.

All of us are born with a fixed number of hair follicles which remain with us—on our heads, in our armpits, on our faces and bodies—for an entire lifetime. Each hair follicle is supplied by one or more oil glands which produce a secretion that gives our hair its richness and gloss. The number of hair follicles—and, therefore, hairs—is inherited. In other words, if your parents had 100,000 hairs on their heads, the chances are that you will have approximately the same number.

Blondes may or may not have more fun than everyone else, but they do have more hair. They average about 120,000 scalp hairs, while brunettes have about 100,000, and redheads only 80,000. But to compensate for this disparity, blonde hairs are thin (fine) and red hairs are thick (coarse). If we weighed the total number of scalp hairs from an average blonde, they would weigh roughly the same as those of a redhead!

Hair loss on the scalp in normal, healthy people varies from about 50 to 120 strands daily, which means that in the course of a year we'll lose about 30,000 scalp hairs from each of our pates. All of these hairs are constantly being replaced, at least until the aging process and certain hormonal changes begin to occur.

Most scalp hairs grow about one-half inch a month, so it takes only two years to grow shoulder-length hair. However, each strand of hair does not grow indefinitely. If you never had your hair cut, your hair would only grow about two and one-half feet. After a period of time (usually two to four years) the hair follicle that produces the individual hair gets tired and stops working. The strand stops growing and eventually falls out, to be replaced by a new "working" hair when the follicle has revived and renewed itself.

Hair grows faster in warm weather, slows down during illness or pregnancy, and falls out more in autumn when "the leaves on the trees begin to drop." Contrary to popular myths and superstitions, hair does not grow thicker or faster when cut or shaved. Nor does it grow after death. And there is no way of telling whether a hair has come from the head of a man or woman.

The following sections cover some basics that can help you have healthier looking hair as well as cope with some common conditions that affect our scalp and hair, such as dandruff, too little hair, and too much hair.

Hair Care

Compare your hair to a woolen sweater. How long would a sweater last if you were to constantly wash, shampoo, comb, brush, color, tint, bleach, tease, straighten, curl, roll, pull, twist, and twirl it? Add to this exposure to the elements: the sun, wind, rain, snow, and sleet and to extremes of heat and cold? How about if you wore it swimming in polluted lakes and streams and chlorinated pools? And then you got it steamed, ironed, sprayed, flipped, oiled, wound, feathered, swirled, dipped, stripped, frosted, perfumed, frizzed, fuzzed, matted, braided, and waxed—and then blown dry by 1200 watts of hot air? How long would it last? A month? A week?

Yet our hair goes through this and more—and, barring certain diseases and conditions, it lasts a lifetime.

Taking good care of your hair, however, can make a big difference in how it looks during its "lifetime": its lustre, its sheen, its body, its "life." And it all begins with shampooing.

The frequency of shampooing is an individual affair. You may shampoo daily or oftener, if need be, without harming the hair or hair follicle in any way.

If your hair is oily or if you live in the city where you are constantly exposed to excessive amounts of dust, grease, grime, soot, and other chemical pollutants, you should shampoo often. And with a good commercial shampoo—not with bar soap.

One of the most important and least stressed facts about shampooing is that in order to derive any benefit from it, the shampoo should be massaged into the entire scalp for *at least 5 minutes*—preferably longer—using fairly hot water. Thorough rinsing is a must. For those who like a cream rinse, I recommend using it in moderation—only small amounts—to prevent the "greasies."

If you blow dry your hair, follow the manufacturer's directions and make sure to keep the blow dryer at least 6 inches away from your hair.

Hair Care Products

There are literally dozens of shampoos flooding the shelves of your drugstore and supermarket. There are shampoos for normal hair, dry hair, and oily hair. For dandruff, psoriasis, eczema. For "thinning" hair. For hair repair. For infants and children. And there are shampoos containing sulfur, salicylic acid, tar, zinc and selenium. Any or all of them may be good. It's basically a matter of choosing one that works for you.

Shampoos

For normal scalp and hair:

Johnson's Baby Shampoo (Johnson & Johnson)
Neutrogena Shampoo (Neutrogena)
Purpose Brand Shampoo (Johnson & Johnson)

For oily scalp and hair:

Pernox Shampoo (Westwood)
Soltex Shampoo (C & M Pharmacal)
Ionil Shampoo (Owen)

For sensitive scalps:

Dara Soapless Shampoo (Owen)

For damaged hair and split ends:

Daragen Shampoo (Owen)
R-Gen Shampoo (Owen)

Cream Rinse

The following is a good cream rinse that many of my patients like:

Ionil Cream Rinse (Owen)

Dandruff

"Nothing stops dandruff like a blue serge suit." If you hadn't heard that one before, well, there is more than a speck of truth to it.

Dandruff is a normal condition. Everybody has it to some degree. It's only when the scaling or flaking that characterizes dandruff becomes excessive—and deposits a fringe on the collar of that dark suit or dress—that we become embarrassed, concerned, and seek medical attention.

To understand dandruff we must know a little about the outer layers of the skin. Like all other cells in the body, skin cells are manufactured to replace those that have outlived their usefulness and died. In the normal skin, the process for a cell to be born, move to the outer edge of the skin surface, and then flake off takes about a month. This constant cycle gives rise to the tiny, scaly flakes that are constantly being shed from the entire skin surface.

On the scalp, this normal, minimal, periodic scaling can usually be controlled by shampooing at frequent intervals with simple, commercial shampoos. In the abnormal process, the cells are born and die at a much faster rate, giving rise to considerable amounts of this flaking which we commonly call dandruff. If the dandruff becomes severe, there may be redness, inflammation, and itching, requiring more than the usual over-the-counter anti-dandruff remedies.

No one really knows why this process occurs. We do know, however, that dandruff does *not* cause baldness, nor does it lead to any serious scalp problem.

Many theories have been proposed regarding the cause of dandruff: hormone imbalance, germs (in the form of bacteria and fungi) living on the scalp, excessive production of oil from the oil glands, dietary indiscretions and deficiencies, allergies, poor hygiene, irritation and inflammation due to various cosmetics and chemicals applied to the scalp, hereditary influences, and emotional stress. Dandruff is rarely seen in children under the age of 12, which leads us to suspect that some type of hormone influences the condition. However, there is no clear-cut proof to substantiate any of these theories.

There are literally dozens of shampoos that are commercially available for the relief of simple dandruff. But remember, there is no *cure* for this condition since a new supply of flakes is produced in about 3 days on everyone's scalp.

And there is no one shampoo that is good for everybody—hence, the large variety and types of products. Your geographic location, the type of water in your home, the mineral content of the water, as well as your particular kind of hair, all play a role in the effectiveness of a particular shampoo.

Traditionally, the medicated shampoos usually contain sulfur, but tar, zinc, selenium, and combinations of these are also popular. Your local pharmacist will have dozens of these preparations for your selection. Find the one you like, the one you feel is most effective, and stick with it.

If your dandruff is persistent and doesn't respond to frequent and conscientious shampooing, check with your physician. You may have psoriasis, eczema, seborrheic dermatitis, or some other condition that requires medical expertise. Be especially watchful if your child has excessive scaling of the scalp, as it is more than likely due to some other type of skin condition.

Treating Dandruff

Shampoos

For the mild to moderate scaling of the scalp—what we ordinarily refer to as dandruff—try any of the following shampoos:

Zincon (Lederle)
Danex (Herbert)
Head & Shoulders (Procter & Gamble)
Selsun Blue (Abbott)
Sebulex Conditioning Shampoo with Protein (Westwood)
Meted Shampoo (Cooper)

For stubborn scaling and itching of the scalp and for conditions such as psoriasis, try a tar shampoo:

T/Gel (Neutrogena)
Polytar (Stiefel)
Sebutone (Westwood)
Zetar (Dermik)
Pentrax (Cooper)
Ionil-T (Owen)
DHS Tar (Persōn & Covey)

Lotion

Or use the following lotion:

Neomark Lotion (C & M Pharmacal)
Directions: Rub into the affected areas at bedtime using a cotton ball.

Hair Dressings

The following are two medicated hair dressings for dandruff and related scaly conditions of the scalp:

Sebucare Lotion (Westwood)
Drest Gel (Dermik)

Male Baldness

Male baldness may be a joke on TV comedy shows, in the flicks, and at cocktail parties, but to those men who cannot adjust to this premature, common hair loss and who literally grasp at every lost hair, it is no joke at all. It can be a source of great anxiety, a personal loss, and a profoundly depressing experience, forcing a man to revise his self-image. To some the Fountain of Youth is no more than a head full of dead, protein threads.

Would it comfort the sufferer to know that Caesar was bald? Does Telly Savalas look as if he's suffering? Mr. Clean?

The hirsute male has forever been a symbol and a proof of virility and physical strength. The biblical Samson, the Greek Hercules, Jupiter, and Neptune were men and gods of prodigious strength and were usually represented as powerful, hairy, and bearded. But so are gorillas!

Male pattern baldness affects well over half the adult male population in the United States and is so common that some degree of hair loss in adult males is considered normal.

Would it console the balding youth to assure him that hair loss has absolutely no adverse effect on virility? Or on potency? Or on strength? The only deleterious effect of premature hair loss is psychological. It may encourage loss of confidence and with it anxiety, stress, and depression.

The cause and extent of male baldness, while not completely understood, are thought to depend on three factors: inheritance, age, and male hormones. If your parents and/or grandparents possessed this bald trait, the chances are that you will inherit it. It is a progressive condition; the older you get, the more hair you will lose.

Would there be any solace in knowing that when you get bald, you lose none of your hair? And that you will go to the grave with the same number of hair follicles with which you were born? What the balding man loses are the longer, darker, coarser hairs which have been replaced with soft, downy fuzz.

Medical science so far has been helpless in reversing, arresting, or curing this pattern. There is, however, a great deal of research going on in an attempt to fatten up and lengthen those downy, vellus hairs.

And, lest you be sadly misled, there presently are no pomades or unguents, no lotions or shampoos, no vitamins or natural food supplements that will grow hair where there are no hair follicles. Hair "restorers" are for the birds—not for the scalp.

It has recently been demonstrated that the female hormone estrogen, when rubbed into the scalp, can lengthen the peach fuzz appreciably and slow down or reduce the rate of pattern baldness. But what about the estrogenic side effect in the male? Do you want larger breasts? A high-pitched voice? A diminished sexual appetite? Think on it...

So what is left for the despondent young man? A hair transplant? A toupee? Or the confidence in knowing that bald may be beautiful. That the highbrow and the egghead—the marks of internal wisdom—are in vogue.

Female Hair Loss

Are American women becoming bald?

There is no clear cut answer to this pressing problem. But we do know that in the past two decades there have been more and more complaints in physicians' offices from women in their 30s and 40s about hair loss —steady, progressive, diffuse, mysterious hair loss. There are very few medical conditions that produce more emotional trauma than the pronounced thinning of scalp hair in young and middle-aged, otherwise healthy females.

Years ago, doctors rarely saw cases of female baldness. But recently, women have begun to notice a gradual, regular, and progressive increase in the number of hairs lost with each brushing and combing—more hair in the wash basin. And, after months or years, a realization that there has occurred visible thinning—a euphemism for baldness.

The healthy scalp loses 50 to 120 hairs daily. This loss, however, is balanced out by continuous regrowth. When the rate of hair loss exceeds the rate of new growth, thinning and balding become apparent.

In most cases there really is not an excessive amount of hair loss, rather an underproduction of new hair. This lack of production of new, viable hair can be due to a dozen different reasons.

The major factors in what the dermatologists term "female pattern baldness" are hormonal imbalance, heredity, and the aging process. Hormonal changes are those which occur after childbirth, at menopause (due to diminished production of female hormones), and with certain types of endocrine tumors and imbalances (thyroid trouble, ovarian problems, and other hormone conditions). Hereditary factors also play a strong role in pattern baldness. If a mother or grandmother had sparse hair, it is likely that the daughter and granddaughter will suffer from the same deficiency.

And, finally, the aging process is a strong factor. After producing for so many decades, the hair follicles become weak, tired, and sluggish. Some of them fade away and produce no more—only one of the prices we must pay for growing old.

Additional causes of thinning and balding in our modern woman are due to environmental changes and the products used for beautification. The following are some examples:

- Mechanical tension and violence on the hair shaft due to new hair styles and cosmetic aids. These cause injury to the hair follicle and, when prolonged, interfere with the circulation of the scalp. Examples here include unusual stretching, pulling, and teasing; brush rollers and curlers; tight, restrictive hair-dos; vigorous combing and brushing; hot combs, braiding, and pony tails. Sharp-toothed nylon and metal combs and brushes also cause mechanical injury to the hair shaft and follicle.

- Excessive chemical exposures associated with hair styling (cold wave solutions, bleaches, hair-straighteners, and the like) and increased exposure to synthetic detergents and other additives in commercial shampoos, dyes, and hair sprays.

- Pollutants in our water supply (pesticides and insecticides), in our air (radioactive fallout and other forms of radiation), in sprays and other inhalants, in our food (dyes, additives, and various drugs and hormones given to cattle and poultry), and increased exposure to dangerous chemicals of all sorts.

- Nutritional deficiencies, such as those seen in "crash-dieters" and those suffering from iron-deficiency anemia.

- Various drugs used to treat cancer and anti-coagulants (blood-thinners) used in heart disease.
- Excessive smoking (a more recent suspect).
- Emotional stress and tension, which are believed to impair the circulation of the hair follicle.

What's a woman to do? Here are a few basic do's and don't's for healthy hair:

- Shampoo your hair regularly (daily, if necessary). Use a good commercial shampoo....one you like.
- If you comb and brush your hair, use only pure bristle brushes and hard rubber combs. Don't use plastic or metal varieties.
- Reduce excessive mechanical manipulation of the hair shaft. Avoid teasing and ratting, vigorous combing and brushing, tight, restrictive hair-dos, tight braids and pony tails, and excessive hot-combing. Hair responds best to gentle care.
- Avoid excessive bleaching, dyeing, and hair-straightening.
- Keep up your general health, avoid crash diets, and cut down on smoking.
- Avoid emotional stress and tension.
- Don't be misled by those advertisements and commercials for potions and unguents that promise to grow hair. There ain't no such animal.
- Finally, if the situation does not improve, see your physician.There may be some infection, hormonal imbalance, or medication you have been taking that might be responsible.

And remember, women don't get bald the way men do. The woman in her 40s may have to get used to a thinner crop than she had in her teens, but it is highly unlikely that she will lose all of her "crowning glory."

Excess Hair

One of the unhappiest women I know is a young lady with an excess amount of dark hair on her upper lip, her chin, and her chest. She is not alone. There are countless thousands of women with the same cosmetic problem: superfluous hair—hair where it doesn't belong; hair that doesn't look sporty in the locker room; hair where nobody wants it.

Exactly what do we mean by excess hair? Not what most people believe.

Excess hair does not mean an increase in the number of hairs. Everyone is born with a fixed number of hairs on his or her body. This is genetically determined (inherited).

Hair grows on every portion of the skin except the palms and soles and a few other small areas. Most of these hairs are of the "peach-fuzz" variety (vellus hairs). Others are of the terminal variety—the long, thicker hairs of the scalp (Lady Godiva, Svengali, Rapunzel), the chest (mostly men), and the pubic region.

What is usually considered as excess hairiness results from the vellus hairs becoming longer, darker, and thicker in areas where one expects to have only peach-fuzz.

While excess hair may be due to many factors, for some groups of people it is the normal state of affairs. People from Southern Europe and Middle-Eastern cultures are much hairier than those from Northern Europe and Scandinavian countries; white people are hairier than black people; and Orientals and American Indians are the least hairy of all.

Above and beyond this normal, constitutional hairy excess, there are those women who exhibit a far greater increase in the length and thickness of hair in certain areas which are usually reserved for the "peach-fuzz" variety: the upper lip, the chin, the sides of the face, the areas around the nipples, and the portion of the abdomen extending from the pubic region to the belly-button. (These are the areas that are normally associated with the male pattern hair growth.) This type of superfluous hair—or hypertrichosis—can be especially damaging psychologically to the young and otherwise confident woman—one of those "thousand natural shocks that flesh is heir to."

The causes of excess hair are many and varied. For those with a moderate degree of hairiness the factors involved may be merely a part of normal growth and development. "Moderate degree," however, is a relative term.

The most common cause of excessive hair growth in females is the aging process, or, as some say euphemistically, the "maturing process." Along about the time of menopause, women become deficient in their production of the female hormone estrogen. The decrease of this hormone gives rise to a relative increase in the male-type hormone (androgen), which is responsible for the slow but inexorable proliferation of thick, dark hairs appearing on the upper lip, chin, and cheeks. And, at the same time, the beginning of the steady thinning of the scalp hair. (In females, it appears that these two processes go hand in hand: more hair on the body, less on the scalp.)

Stress and tension can play a role in excess hair growth as well. The hair follicles are under the influence of various hormones and chemicals produced by the body. Emotional tension and stress often lead to a disturbance in the delicate balance of these hormones and chemicals which, in turn, can result in a stimulation of the hair follicle leading to excess hair—not, however, on the head. These hormonal imbalances can also arise in connection with tumors and cysts of the female reproductive organs (ovaries), diseases of the adrenal glands, and abnormal functioning and tumors of other hormone-secreting glands, such as the thyroid or pituitary.

In addition, various drugs and medications can occasionally produce hypertrichosis when given over a period of time. These include drugs for epilepsy (Dilantin), cortisone-like drugs, and a host of others.

Treatment for Excess Hair

Women who have excessive hair—on the body or the face—can suffer deep embarrassment, even torment. It isn't something you get rid of by saying "presto," but there are ways to deal with the problem.

A wag once said that the only answer to hirsutism (superfluous hair) is the impractical one of choosing one's parents. (This can also be said of baldness!)

The concealment or removal of excess hair in an otherwise normal woman (that is, a woman who has no severe hormonal disease or disturbance) can be accomplished in a number of ways: bleaching, shaving, plucking with tweezers, depilatory creams and lotions, waxes, abrasive applicators, and electrolysis. All have their drawbacks, and all, except electrolysis, are temporary measures.

Bleaching: Bleaching with commercially available products can conceal excessive, fine, fuzzy hair growth on the upper lip and forearms. It is most effective for small amounts of unwanted hair.

When done properly, bleaching is simple, safe and painless. Repeated use of bleaching agents, however, can damage the hair shaft and cause temporary breakage. It can also irritate the skin. If you do use a bleach and develop a rash, try a different product.

Shaving: There is a popular misconception that shaving or cutting your hair makes it grow faster, thicker, coarser, and darker. There is no scientific evidence to support this belief. (If this were true, there would be very few bald men!)

The portion of hair emerging from the surface of the skin is non-living—a dead protein thread. Cutting your hair cannot influence the growing portion of the hair, which is embedded in the hair follicle beneath the surface of the skin. It is, however, a temporary measure and must be repeated fairly often to avoid the stubbly feel and the "5 o'clock shadow" look.

If you shave with a safety razor, I recommend a clean, single track blade. (Refrain from using an old, used, ragged blade.) The women in my household swear by the Flicker, an ingenious, disposable device which shaves hair swiftly and painlessly. Do not shave too closely as this practice may lead to ingrown hairs. It is also advisable to shave *with* the grain, not against it.

If you use an electric shaver, try a pre-shave lotion. You'll find that shaving is easier, and you'll be less likely to nick the skin.

Plucking (Tweezing): Plucking out hairs with tweezers is a popular and effective, although somewhat painful, way to remove temporarily scattered hairs on the face, chest, and eyebrows. Because of the discomfort and irritation, this method should be reserved for small areas of excess hair.

Plucking has no adverse side effects and, as with other methods of temporary hair removal, will not cause the hairs to grow faster, coarser, or darker. Constant and repeated tweezing in the same area, however, may cause tiny, pitted scars.

When using the plucking method, make sure the skin and the tweezers are scrupulously clean to avoid infection. Also, *do not* pluck hairs from moles, warts, or other tumors. This can cause disagreeable side effects in the form of bleeding, infection, and change in the type of cell growth.

Hint: applying an ice cube to the area just before plucking may minimize the pain.

Chemical Depilatories: Available in creams, liquids, and foams, these products are made up of chemicals which weaken the hairs, causing them to break off or dissolve just below the surface of the skin. This is one of the best, easiest, and most popular methods for temporary hair removal of unwanted hair on the arms, legs and underarm areas. One word of caution: *do not* use these products on broken or abraded skin.

The first time you use a chemical depilatory, try it on a "test" area first to make sure your skin isn't overly sensitive to it. Then wash and dry the area to be depilated. Apply the chemical and leave it on for a specific length of time—usually 10 or 15 minutes, depending on the directions given by the manufacturer. (If you leave it on longer than recommended, it can severely irritate your skin.) Then wash the area with soap and water and pat it dry. You may then want to apply a soothing, emollient cream or lotion, as the chemical may dry out your skin.

Waxing: One of the oldest and least popular methods of temporary hair removal is molten wax. Hot, melted wax is poured onto the skin, left to cool and solidify, and then rapidly stripped off. The hairs which have been embedded in the wax are plucked out as the wax is removed.

This type of hair removal is longer-lasting than some of the other methods described, as it takes about 4 to 6 weeks for waxed hair to grow back. However, there is always some degree of pain and skin irritation.

Abrasives: Pumice stones have been used for centuries to "wear off" excess hair. Although simple and inexpensive, this method of hair removal is rather tedious and uncomfortable and, therefore, not suitable for large areas.

Electrolysis: There is only one safe way to remove excess hair permanently: destroying the hair root with an electric current. This is known as electrolysis.

Performed by a physician or trained electrologist, electrolysis consists of inserting a fine platinum or steel wire needle into the opening of the hair follicle. An electric current, transmitted down the needle, permanently destroys the hair root. Once the root is destroyed, the hair can no longer grow back.

While several types of electric current may be used, the basic procedure is the same. The results will depend upon the skill of the operator. Even in the most competent hands, however, electrolysis is a long, expensive, and tedious process. It is also somewhat painful, particularly on areas other than the face.

Electrolysis is most effective for the coarse, darker hairs, not the fine, "peach-fuzz," lanugo-type hairs. It has no effect on the cause of excessive hair growth. All it can do is destroy the existing hair.

Electrolysis is not 100% effective, and repeated treatments are often necessary to destroy successfully all the unwanted hairs. There are several reasons for this. Some hair follicles may be bent or crooked. The electrical current for the particular follicle may be insufficient (the higher the current, the greater the pain; therefore, the operator tries to "get away" with the smallest current that might do the job). Also, since the electrologist works below the surface of the skin, the insertion of the needle into the hair follicle is essentially a blind procedure, and, therefore, cannot be performed with absolute certainty. Another common occurrence is that the hair will come out, but the papilla (the hair root) will not have been destroyed, resulting in the regrowth of that particular hair. Thus, depending upon the skill of the operator and the nature of the hair being treated, a single strand may have to be treated several times before it stops growing. Coarse hairs may return three of four times, but these become finer at each regrowth, and eventually the root is so effectively destroyed that the hairs can no longer grow.

"Sittings" with the electrologist should be no longer than half an hour during which only a limited number of hairs (about 50) should be removed. To avoid excessive inflammation, those hairs lying close together should not be dealt with at the same time. Also, the skin and needles must be adequately sterilized to prevent infection.

In the hands of a competent, well-trained, and conscientious electrologist, the dangers and side effects are minimal. Occasionally, scarring and fine pits will develop in places formerly occupied by hairs. (This is seen more commonly on the upper lip.) In addition, excessive pigmentation may develop, but this is rare and usually quickly disappears. Since it is impossible to predict the nature of scarring or healing in any given patient, the electrologist should try a small trial area first and check the results.

I do not recommend the small, battery-operated, do-it-yourself kits. It is virtually impossible for a person to insert a tiny needle into a hair follicle on his or her face—while looking in a mirror! And when improperly used, these treatments can lead to irreparable scarring.

For those who are contemplating electrolysis, don't expect too much—the average patient quickly tires of the experience and the cost. Because only a small percentage of hairs can be removed at one sitting and because some regrowth of hair—even in the most skilled hands—will always recur after electrolysis, it requires firm determination on the part of both operator and patient. A severe case of excess hair (hirsutism) may require years of treatment.

But despite its limitations, in selected patients electrolysis has been found to be useful and successful.

Alopecia Areata

It goes by the lilting name of alopecia areata, but patchy hair loss—as it's commonly called—would not be desirable by any name. Still, it can be treated, so don't despair.

Patchy hair loss is pretty much what it says it is—a condition of the scalp and other hairy areas of the body that begins with the sudden appearance of one or more small, round or oval, bald patches which gradually enlarge over a period of weeks. It affects all age groups but is more common among children and young adults.

The bald patches appear rather quickly on an otherwise normal, healthy, hairy area. They do not itch, burn, or cause any pain. The scalp is the area most commonly affected, but alopecia areata can affect the beard, eyebrows, eyelashes, and any other hairy region as well. The hairs at the periphery of these balding patches are usually loose and easily pulled out.

In severe cases, patches on the scalp become so large that they merge to produce a total loss of all the scalp hair. This is known as alopecia totalis. In exceptional cases, the condition may progress until every hair of the entire body is lost. This is known as alopecia universalis. (Queen Elizabeth I of England contracted this condition in 1562 following her severe bout with smallpox. She was completely bald for the remainder of her life and resorted to wigs and other artifices.)

Why, on some people, the hair root simply stops making hair is not known. However, it has been associated with certain hormonal changes, with blows to the head, and, frequently, with severe emotional strain or shock.

In some cases other members of the immediate family are similarly affected.

Basically, alopecia areata is a temporary, self-limiting disease. In many cases, even without treatment, the hairs begin to grow back slowly, after a few weeks or months. The course is erratic and unpredictable, but, as a rule of thumb, the greater the initial hair loss and the earlier in life it begins, the more likely it is to persist or recur.

At first, the regrowth is in the form of fine, downy, white hairs. Eventually these hairs develop their normal texture and color.

Is there any treatment for alopecia areata? Yes.

First of all, stop worrying. Make sure your general health is not impaired. Only your general physician can correct any deficiencies and give you a "clean bill of health."

More specific types of treatment include injections of certain cortisone-like drugs directly into the bald patches. These are relatively painless and can hasten the regrowth and often prevent further hair loss. In severe cases, applying cortisone-type creams to the patches and covering them tightly with plastic or Saran Wrap may help.

Massage and hair tonics are worthless. If they do seem to help, it is only because time itself has allowed nature to do its job.

If you have an extensive and persistent case of alopecia areata, you may find that a hairpiece will give you peace of mind.

9 Treatment Summary

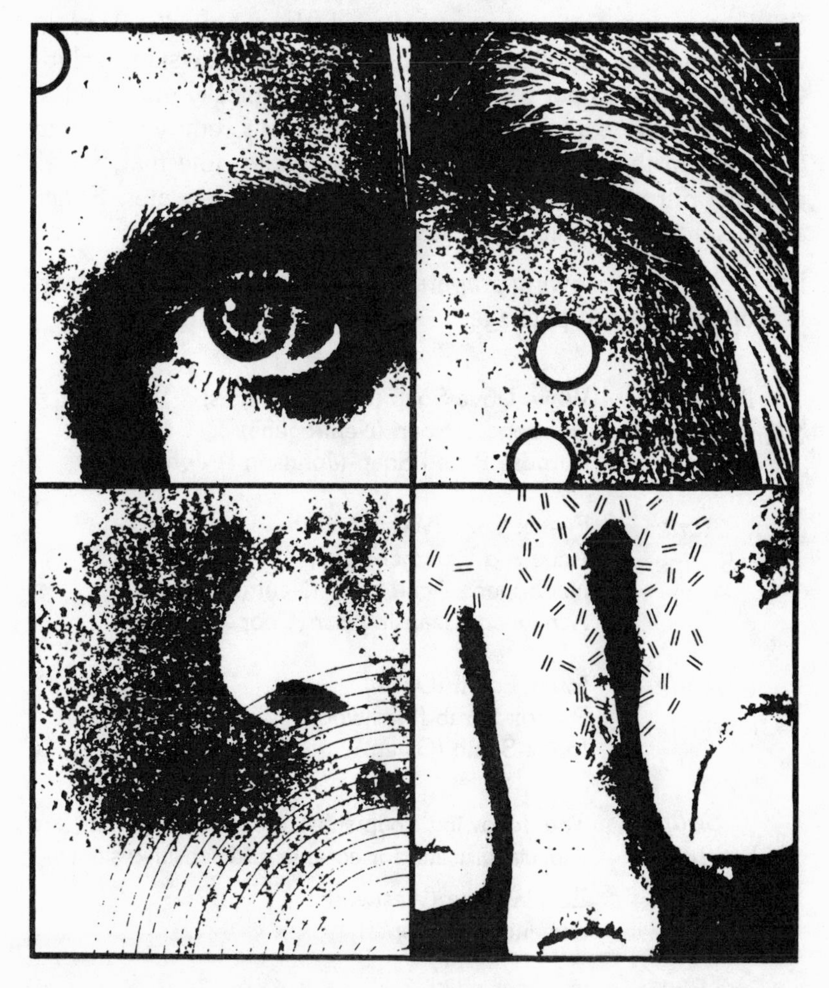

The following information is a compilation of the nearly 200 "drugs and devices" that have been mentioned in the previous chapters. It gives directions on how each is to be used, what to ask your pharmacist to compound for you, and the names of the pharmaceutical companies that manufacture the "ready-made" preparations.

Soaps & Cleansers

Soaps and cleansers are products which, when dissolved in water, can break up oil and dirt on the surface of the skin. Included here are detergent bars which, while chemically unrelated to soap, have the same function and action—to remove dirt and grease from the skin. It might be of interest to note that, for all practical purposes, the primary cleansing agent is water. Soaps and detergents merely help the water do a better job.

For each of the following preparations, follow the directions clearly marked on each package.

Normal Skin Soaps	White Dove Soap (Lever Brothers) Neutrogena Soap (Neutrogena) Purpose Brand Soap (Johnson & Johnson)
Acne Soaps	Fostex Cake (Westwood) Acne-Aid Detergent Soap (Stiefel) Neutrogena Acne Soap (Neutrogena) Acnaveen Cleansing Bar (Cooper)
Acne Cleansers	Ionax Foam (Owen) Pernox Scrub (Westwood) Ionax Scrub (Owen)
Soap Substitutes	The following soap-substitute cleansing bars are especially useful for eczema and sensitive skin: Lowila Cake (Westwood) Aveenobar (Cooper)
Dry Skin Soaps	The following are superfatted soaps which help moisturize dry skin: Oilatum Soap (Stiefel) Alpha Keri Soap (Westwood) Neutrogena Dry Skin Soap (Neutrogena) Emulave (Cooper)

Basis Soap (Beiersdorf)

Psoriasis Soaps

Polytar Soap (Stiefel)
Packer's Pine Tar Soap (Cooper)

Antibacterial Soaps

To prevent bacterial buildup, the following soaps have antibacterial properties:

Dial Soap (Armour)
Safeguard Soap (Procter & Gamble)
Hibiclens (Stuart)

"Degreasing" Cleansers

The following liquid preparations are good "degreasing" cleansers for acne:

Drytex (C & M Pharmacal)
Ionax Astringent Cleanser (Owen)
Seba-Nil Liquid Cleanser (Owen)

Drying Pads

These drying pads help dry up acne and oily skin:

Seba-Nil Towelettes (Owen)
Stri-Dex Pads (Lehn & Fink)

Compresses, Soaks, & Wet Dressings

Compresses, soaks, and wet dressings all mean essentially the same thing to the physician. They are variations of the mildest form of dermatologic therapy and are used in localized skin disorders to soothe and reduce inflammation (as in hives and insect bites); to cleanse and dry up acute, weeping and oozing dermatoses (as in eczema and poison ivy dermatitis); to cool painful areas of the skin (as in sunburn); and to destroy germs of infected, crusted lesions (as in impetigo and infected athlete's foot).

The following information includes several recommended preparations as well as general instructions for applying compresses, soaks, and wet dressings.

Preparations

AluWets Wet Dressing Crystals (Stiefel)

Directions: Dissolve one packet in 12 ounces of warm water. For larger volumes, use the same proportions (e.g., 2 packets to 24 ounces, 3 packets to 36 ounces).

Domeboro Powder Packets (Dome)

Directions: Dissolve one packet in one pint (16 oz.) of warm water. For larger volumes, use proportionately.

Bluboro Powder (Herbert)

Directions: Same as for Domeboro Powder above.

Dalidome Powder Packets (Dome)

Directions: Same as for Domeboro Powder above.

Salt solution

Directions: Dissolve one teaspoon of table salt in one pint of warm water.

Milk (preferably whole milk)

Directions: Remove milk from the refrigerator and let stand for about 15 minutes.

How to apply compresses, soaks and wet dressings:

Localized Areas

For localized areas of skin disorders (except areas on the hands and feet), the proper way to apply compresses or wet dressings is as follows:

Use either a folded cotton handkerchief, pieces of bed linen, or old shirting or sheeting folded 8-ply. Dip this into the solution you prepared and gently wring it out so that the cloth is sopping wet. Pat this on the affected area—on and off, on and off—remoistening the cloth when necessary. Do this for 10 or 15 minutes every hour or so until the lesions have cooled down, have begun to dry, or until the crusts have been removed. After compressing, pat the area dry. When the lesions have become sufficiently dry, you may apply a lotion or cream appropriate for the condition. (If you plan to use the same cloth for compresses later, make sure to rinse it out in plain water to eliminate any chemical build-up in the material.)

Hands

For acute, weeping dermatoses of the fingers and hands, the proper and most efficient way to "soak" these areas is as follows:

Buy 2 or 3 pairs of Dermal Gloves. (You can buy these at your drugstore.) With the gloves on, immerse your hands in the appropriate solution (see previous section) and remove them every 3 or 4 seconds: in and out, in and out. Keep up this procedure for 10 or 15 minutes and then remove the gloves. (Never let the gloves dry on the hands!) Pat dry.

Repeat this procedure every hour or two until the oozing, weeping or crusting have begun to dry up. At bedtime, apply the recommended cream or lotion or paste and wear the gloves to bed.

Feet

For acute weeping disorders of the feet and toe webs, obtain a plastic basin that holds about a gallon of liquid. Put a large turkish towel under the basin. Put on soft, white, cotton socks. If your toes are affected, keep them separated with lamb's wool or one inch squares of old cotton sheeting or shirting (*not cotton balls*). Then follow these steps:

Fill the basin with the solution (see previous section). Immerse your feet in the basin. Count till five. Take the right foot out and place on the towel. Count till five. Put the right foot back in the basin. Count till five. Take the left foot out and place on the towel. Count till five. Put the left foot back in the basin. Count till five. Take the right foot out and place on the towel, etc.

Repeat this procedure for 20 to 30 minutes. (This can be done while watching your favorite TV show or reading.) Try to keep the water warm by every so often adding hot water to the solution. At no time should you allow the socks to dry on your feet. After you have completed the soaking process, remove the socks (and lamb's wool) and dry the feet thoroughly.

Repeat the entire process every 3 or 4 hours until the weeping and oozing have stopped. At bedtime apply the recommended cream or paste and put on a clean pair of white cotton socks.

If your toe webs are affected, as in athlete's foot, always keep them separated by means of lamb's wool or cotton material. Always means 24 hours a day.

Baths

Medicated baths are useful in managing widespread and generalized rashes. A convenient method of applying medication to the entire skin surface, baths soothe, soften, reduce inflammation, and relieve itching and dryness. The best temperature for a medicated bath is 100° to 114°F (40° to 44°C).

Anti-Itch Baths

The following preparations can soothe and lubricate dry skin and combat itching. Fill the tub about half full of warm (tepid) water and add any of the following:

Alpha Keri Therapeutic Bath Oil (Westwood)

Directions: Add 2 to 4 capfuls to the tub and soak for 20 to 30 minutes. (*Caution:* Guard against slipping in the tub!)

Lubath (Parke-Davis)

Directions: The same as for Alpha Keri Bath Oil.

nutraSpa Bath Oil (Owen)
Directions: The same as for Alpha Keri Bath Oil.

Surfol Post-Immersion Bath Oil (Stiefel)
Directions: See directions on the label.

Aveeno Oilated Bath (Cooper)
Directions: See directions on the label.

Tar Baths

Baths containing derivatives of tar are helpful in such widespread, scaly conditions as psoriasis, eczema, lichen planus, and other generalized dermatoses. They also help relieve the itching accompanying these disorders.

Balnetar (Westwood)
Directions: Add 2 to 4 capfuls to a tub of warm water and soak for 20 to 30 minutes. (*Caution:* Guard against slipping in the tub!)

Polytar Bath Oil (Stiefel)
Directions: The same as for Balnetar.

Lavatar (Doak)
Directions: The same as for Balnetar.

Lotions

Lotions used for the treatment of skin disorders fall into 2 main categories: "shake" lotions and "creamy-type" lotions, also called emulsions or liniments.

"Shake" Lotions

Shake lotions are suspensions of powder in water which require shaking before being applied. (Calamine lotion is the prime example of a shake lotion.) As the lotion evaporates, it tends to cool and soothe. When it dries, it leaves a protective film of powder on the skin. Medicated ingredients are often incorporated into lotions to give them anti-itch and healing properties.

Anti-Itch Lotions

The following lotions are inexpensive, easy to apply and particularly suited for widespread and extensive itchy eruptions, such as poison ivy dermatitis, eczema and acute sun-poisoning.

Calamine Lotion (USP)

Directions: Apply to affected areas 3 or 4 times daily using your fingers or a soft, one inch, flat varnish paint brush.

Or ask your pharmacist to make up the following:

Phenol	½%
Calamine Lotion (USP)	to make 4 oz.

Directions: The same as for calamine lotion.

The following preparation has an added anti-itch ingredient (menthol) which is cooling as well. It can be used for moderately severe itching. Ask your pharmacist to compound this for you:

Menthol	¼%
Phenol	½%
Calamine Lotion (USP)	to make 4 oz.

Directions: The same as for calamine lotion.

Acne Lotions

For mild acne try any of the following lotions and apply to the affected zits at bedtime:

Fostril Lotion (Westwood)
Acne-Aid Lotion (Stiefel)
Komed Lotion (mild) (Barnes-Hind)

For moderately severe acne try:

Benoxyl 5 Lotion (Stiefel)
Vanoxide Lotion (Dermik)
Persadox Lotion 5% (Owen)

For more severe acne, when the pimples are stubborn and are not relieved by above medications, try one of the following:

Benoxyl 10 Lotion (Stiefel)
Persadox HP Lotion (Owen)

Cold Sore Lotions

Apply any of the following to the cold sores every 3 to 4 hours:

Campho-Phenique Liquid (Glenbrook)
Cold Sore Lotion (DeWitt)

Lotions for Dandruff & Itchy Scalp

Sebucare Lotion (Westwood)
Directions: Massage into scalp daily.

Neomark Lotion (C & M Pharmacal)
Directions: Apply to the scalp at bedtime.

Lotion for Psoriasis of Scalp

Neomark Lotion (C&M Pharmacal)
Directions: Rub into scalp at night using a cotton ball.

"Creamy" Lotions (Emulsions or Liniments)

These preparations are soothing, less drying, and more elegant in appearance than shake lotions. They are smoother, more creamy, and almost vanish into the skin.

Anti-Itch Lotions

Rhulicort Lotion (Lederle)
Directions: Apply to itchy areas 3 or 4 times daily.

Schamberg's Lotion (C&M Pharmacal)
Directions: Same as above.

Or ask your pharmacist to compound one of the following:

Menthol	¼%
Phenol	½%

Calamine Liniment (USP)	to make 8 oz.

Directions: Apply to itchy areas 3 or 4 times daily.

Menthol	¼%
Phenol	½%
Mī-Skin Lotion	to make 4 oz.

Directions: Apply as above.

Dry Skin Lotions

Simple emollients for softening and lubricating the skin to keep it smooth, pliable, resilient and elastic:

Keri Lotion (Westwood)
Neutrogena Lotion (Neutrogena)
Mī-Skin Lotion (Michel)
Nutraderm Lotion (Owen)
Lubriderm Lotion (Parke-Davis)
Shepard's Cream Lotion (Dermik)
Wibi Dry Skin Lotion (Owen)
Nivea Creme Lotion (Beiersdorf)

Dry Skin & Anti-Itch Lotions

The following preparations have a softening and moisturizing effect on the skin and, in addition, help relieve the itching that is often associated with dry skin:

Carmol-10 Lotion (Syntex)
LactiCare Lotion (Stiefel)
Nutraplus Lotion (Owen)
Aquacare/HP Lotion (Herbert)

The following is a moisturizing lotion that won't cause acne:

Aquaderm (C & M Pharmacal)

Creams

Creams are suspensions of oil in water that are used to carry active medicaments into the skin. They are soft preparations which spread thinly and vanish into the skin and, thus, are cosmetically more acceptable and more elegant than ointments and pastes. By accommodating different ingredients, creams can be used for a number of skin disorders.

Acne Creams

Acne-Aid Cream (Stiefel)—for mild acne
Persadox HP Cream (Owen)—for stubborn acne

Directions for both: Apply to the pimples at bedtime.

Moisturizing Cream

The following is a moisturizing cream that won't cause acne:

T&C Therapeutic Moisturizing Face Cream (Dermalab)

Athlete's Foot Creams

Tinactin Cream (Schering)

Directions: Apply to feet and toe webs twice daily.

Vioform Cream 3% (Ciba)

Directions: Same as for Tinactin Cream.

Creams for Very Dry Skin

Carmol-20 Cream (Syntex)
Purpose Dry Skin Cream (Johnson & Johnson)

Directions for both: Apply 2 or 3 times daily.

Anti-Itch Creams

For insect bites, lichen planus, hives, chronic eczema, etc., use the following:

Rhulicort Cream (Lederle)

Or have your pharmacist compound the following:

Menthol	1/4%
Phenol	1/2%
Cold cream	to make 2 oz.

Directions: Apply for itching 2 or 3 times daily.

Creams for Rectal Itch

For rectal itching try either of the following:

Rhulicort Cream (Lederle)

Vioform Cream 3% (Ciba)

Directions for both: Apply every 3 or 4 hours and after each bowel movement.

Or have your pharmacist compound the following:

Menthol	0.1%
Phenol	¼%
Cold cream	to make 2 oz.

Direction: Apply to rectal area 2 or 3 times daily and after each bowel movement.

Creams for Psoriasis

With tar:

Alphosyl Cream (Reed and Carnrick)
Pragmatar (SKF)
Tegrin (Block)

Directions for all of the above: Apply to the affected areas twice daily.

With salicylic acid (compounded preparation):

Salicylic acid	3%
Cold cream	to make 4 oz.

Directions: Apply to affected areas twice daily.

Ointments

Ointments are greasy and occlusive preparations. By incorporating active medications into them, they are useful in chronic, dry, scaly, thick, and stubborn skin disorders. They can help remove crusts and scales and are useful in softening dry, flaky skin. They are, however, somewhat messy to use.

Antibacterial Ointments

The following ointments are good for impetigo and other bacterial infections of the skin:

Mycitracin Ointment (Upjohn)

Directions: Apply to the affected areas 4 times daily.

Neosporin Ointment (Burroughs Wellcome)
Directions: Same as above.

Antifungal Ointments

These antifungal ointments can be used for athlete's foot and other ringworm infections:

Vioform Ointment 3% (Ciba)
Directions: Apply to the affected areas twice daily.

Or have your pharmacist compound the following:

Whitfield's Ointment (one-half strength)
Directions: Same as above.

Ointment for Cold Sores

Blistex Ointment (Blistex)
Directions: Apply to cold sores 3 or 4 times daily.

Ointment for Molluscum Contagiosum

5% Ammoniated Mercury Ointment (Lilly)
Directions: Apply to affected areas twice daily.

Pastes

Pastes are preparations that have about 50% powdered ingredients in a greasy base, such as petrolatum. They work to protect the skin from outside forces, such as rubbing or scratching; they absorb moisture; and they help dry up weeping and oozing lesions. Since they tend to "stay put," they help to carry active medicated ingredients to the areas where they are needed. Unfortunately, they also are somewhat messy. They usually require bandaging, and they can be difficult to remove.

The best way to apply pastes is with a wooden applicator, such as a doctor's tongue depressor. They should be left on all day long. To remove pastes, use a light mineral oil or vegetable oil.

Protective Paste

Zinc Oxide (Lassar's) Paste (USP)
Directions: Apply to affected areas once or twice

daily. Apply one layer on top of the other.

This is unquestionably the best and cheapest preparation to protect against diaper rash, to soothe painful cold sores of the genital region, and to protect against sunburn and sun poisoning. Cosmetically inelegant, it serves its purpose as no other preparation of its kind can do.

Paste for Rectal Itch

Ask your pharmacist to make the following preparation:

Menthol	0.1%
Phenol	¼%
Burow's Solution	10cc
Aquaphor	20gm
Paste of Zinc Oxide	to make 2 oz.

Directions: Apply 2 or 3 times daily and after each bowel movement.

Gels

Gels are colorless and transparent preparations. They liquify on contact with the skin and dry as thin, greaseless, non-staining films.

Acne Gels

Transact Gel (Westwood)—for mild acne

Neutrogena Acne Drying Gel (Neutrogena)—for mild acne

Fostex BPO Antibacterial Acne Gel (Westwood)—for stubborn acne

Directions for all of the above: Apply to the affected pimples at bedtime.

Anti-Itch Gel

For itching caused by insect bites, hives, lichen planus, etc., use the following:

Topic (Syntex)

Directions: Rub in gently every 3 or 4 hours.

Gel for Dandruff

Drest Gel (Dermik)
Directions: Apply to scalp once daily.

Gels for Psoriasis

The following gels contain tar for the treatment of psoriasis:

Estar Gel (Westwood)
psoriGel (Owen)
Directions: Rub in gently twice daily.

Gel for Canker Sores

Proxigel (Reed and Carnrick)
Directions: Massage on to affected areas 2 or 3 times daily.

Gel for Cold Sores

Resolve (Dow)
Directions: Apply to cold sores 3 or 4 times daily.

Varnishes

Varnishes are solutions of active medications that evaporate rapidly and deposit the active ingredients in a fine adherent film (like clear nail polish).

Varnishes for Warts

Compound W Wart Remover (Whitehall)
Directions: Apply to warts at bedtime.

Wart-Away (The DePree Company)
Directions: Same as above.

Compounded preparations:

Salicylic acid	10%
Lactic acid	10%
Flexible Collodion	to make ½ oz.

Directions: Ask your pharmacist to dispense this in

an amber bottle with a glass-rod applicator. Apply to warts at bedtime.

Varnish for Molluscum Contagiosum		
	Salicylic acid	5%
	Lactic acid	5%
	Flexible Collodion	to make ½ oz.

Directions: Apply to tops of each lesion at bedtime.

Shampoos

A shampoo is little more than a dilute solution of soap or detergent used for washing the hair and scalp. Colors, perfumes, and other additives merely increase the price; they do not necessarily add to the effectiveness of the preparation.

For Normal Hair

Johnson's Baby Shampoo (Johnson & Johnson)
Purpose Brand Shampoo (Johnson & Johnson)
Neutrogena Shampoo (Neutrogena)

For Oily Hair

Pernox Shampoo (Westwood)
Ionil Shampoo (Owen)
Soltex Shampoo (C&M Pharmacal)

Dandruff Shampoos

Meted Shampoo (Cooper)
Zincon Shampoo (Lederle)
Danex Shampoo (Herbert)
Sebulex Conditioning Shampoo with Protein (Westwood)
Head & Shoulders Shampoo (Procter & Gamble)
Selsun Blue (Abbott)

Tar Shampoo

The following shampoos for excess dandruff, psoriasis and other stubborn, scaly conditions of the scalp contain tar which may stain blonde or grey hair.

T/Gel Shampoo (Neutrogena) (no tar odor)
Polytar Shampoo (Stiefel)
Sebutone Shampoo (Westwood)
Zetar Shampoo (Dermik)
Pentrax Shampoo (Cooper)
DHS Tar Shampoo (Persōn and Covey)
Ionil-T Shampoo (Owen)
Vanseb-T Shampoo (Herbert)

Damaged Hair

Daragen Shampoo (Owen)
R-Gen Shampoo (Owen)

Sensitive Scalps

Dara Soapless Shampoo (Owen)

Lice

Vonce Shampoo (Unipharm)
Directions: Follow directions on the bottle.

Cream Rinse

Ionil Cream Rinse (Owen)

Sun-Protective Agents

Depending on their levels of melanin pigmentation, people have been classified into various skin types. Depending upon the type of skin you have, there is a wide range of sunscreen products that have been rated according to the degree of protection they can give against ultraviolet radiation. This rating is known as the Sun Protection Factor (SPF).

Skin Type I

These people are fair-skinned and fair-haired and may have freckles. These people are advised to use sunsceens with a Sun Protection Factor of 10 to 15:

PreSun 15 (Westwood)
Total Eclipse (Herbert)
Super Shade (Plough)
Pabanol (Elder)

Solbar Plus 15 (Persōn & Covey)

Skin Type II These people are fair-skinned but not as sensitive to the sun's rays as those of Type I. These people are advised to use sunscreens with an SPF of 6 to 10:

PreSun 8 (Westwood)
Eclipse (Herbert)

Skin Type III These people have darker skin and usually tan but sometimes burn. These people are advised to use sunscreens with an SPF of 4 to 6:

PreSun 4 (Westwood)
Partial Eclipse (Herbert)
Solbar (Persōn and Covey)
Sundown (Johnson & Johnson)

Skin Type IV These people always tan well and almost never develop sunburn. They may use sunscreens with an SPF of 2 to 4:

Sundare (Cooper)
RVP (Elder)

Sun Block The following is an excellent, inexpensive, although cosmetically-inelegant sun-blocking agent that mechanically blocks out all the harmful rays of the sun:

Zinc Oxide Paste

Lipsticks The following sun-blocking "lipsticks" protect the delicate areas of the lips:

PreSun Sunscreen Lip Protection (Westwood)
Eclipse Sunscreen Lip and Face Protectant (Herbert)
Sun Stick (Cooper)
RVPaba Lipstick (Elder)

Make-ups

Women with normal skin—that is, skin that is problem-free—can usually wear any kind of make-up. Those make-ups, however, that contain lanolin and other greasy and oily ingredients often cause a plugging-up of the oil glands of the face and can produce acne lesions in women who never had an acne problem before.

Acne Make-ups

The following are non-medicated make-ups—oil-free and water-based—that are recommended to prevent acne lesions:

Clinique: Pore Minimizer
Revlon: Touch and Glow
Estée Lauder: Fresh Air
Ultima: Skim Milk
Revlon: Moon Drops

Non-medicated Make-ups

A few pharmaceutical companies also manufacture an entire line of non-medicated make-ups. These can be purchased in all well-stocked drugstores and in many good department stores. They include the following:

Allercreme Hypo-Allergenic Cosmetics (Owen)
Almay Hypo-allergenic Cosmetics
Ar-Ex Products Company
Marcelle

Medicated Make-ups

Liquimat Lotion (Owen)
Clearasil Regular Tinted Cream (Vick Chemical)
Acnotex Lotion (C&M Pharmacal)

Dyes & Stains

The following preparations are used to cover up, mask, or color vitiligo (depigmented) lesions to the natural tone of the surrounding skin:

Dy-O-Derm (Owen)
Directions: Apply as directed on the label.

Vitadye (Elder)
Directions: Apply as directed on the label.

Cover-up

Covermark (Lydia O'Leary) (in 8 shades)
Note: This is an opaque cream that conceals blemishes and covers up the light areas of vitiligo. It is available in most large department stores.

Antihistamines

Antihistamines are useful in controlling the itching of certain skin disorders, mainly the itching associated with hives. It is important to note that there are certain undesirable side effects associated with these substances, not the least of which is drowsiness. If you contemplate driving, or if other activities require that you be mentally alert, avoid using antihistamines. Also, do not take them in combination with alcoholic beverages or sleeping pills and do not take them during pregnancy. (Other cautions should appear on the label of each bottle. If they do not, ask your pharmacist to let you see them.)

The following are only a few of the over-the-counter antihistamines:

Tablets

Chlor-Trimeton Tablets 4mg (Schering)
Adult dose: One tablet every 4 hours for itching. Since these tablets are scored (marked with a groove down the middle), they may be broken in half to adjust the dose.

Dimetane Tablets 4mg (Robins)
Adult dose: One tablet every 4 hours for itching.

Syrup

Chlor-Trimeton Syrup (Schering)
Child dose: Use one-half to one teaspoonful every 4 hours for itching. One teaspoonful equals 2 mg of Chlor-Trimeton.

Miscellaneous Skin Care Aids

There are countless other products which can be useful in the treatment and prevention of skin disease. The following are just a few miscellaneous skin care products.

Foot Powder

The following dusting powder helps keep feet and toe webs dry:

Zeasorb Powder (Stiefel)

Note: This helps protect the feet against such conditions as athlete's foot, contact dermatitis of the feet, and excessive sweating of the feet and toes.

Anal Cleanser

Balneol (Geigy)
This is a soothing, emollient preparation for **cleansing** the **anal area**. It helps relieve itching and, by providing a soothing, protective film, helps stop irritation due to toilet tissue.

Cold sore Preparation

Use the following preparation for **cold sores**:

Camphor Spirit (N.F.)

Apply with a cotton swab to affected areas 3 or 4 times daily.

Lamb's Wool

Use **lamb's wool** to keep your toes separated in conditions such as weeping and oozing "athlete's foot," contact dermatitis of the feet and toes, eczema, etc.

Dermal Gloves

Use **Dermal Gloves** for soaking your hands in special solutions when treating acute dermatoses of the fingers and hands. They can also be used as cotton liners *under* cotton-lined rubber gloves, for those people who have chronic hand eczemas and who have to do "wet work," such as laundry and dishes, etc.

Meat Tenderizer A mixture of half unseasoned **meat tenderizer** and half water will give much relief when applied early to insect bites and stings.

Adhesive Tape One-inch wide Johnson & Johnson Zonas **adhesive** tape can be used for warts on fingers and around and under nails.

Ice Cubes **Ice cubes** are useful in aborting early cold sores. You can also use them to relieve insect bites and stings.

Whole Milk **Whole milk**, removed from the refrigerator and allowed to stand for 10 to 15 minutes, can be used in compresses for acute, painful and oozing conditions (such as cold sores) of the lips, genital and rectal areas.

Index

K

L

M

M (cont.)

N

O

P

P (cont.)

P (cont.)

Q

R

S

S (cont.)

S (cont.)

T

I will be glad to answer any special question you may have regarding a particular skin condition or its treatment. Use the space below to type or clearly print your question. Please limit your question to no more than 100 words. Enclose a self-addressed, stamped, business envelope with your request and allow six to eight weeks for a reply.

Your Name ______________________

Address ______________________
street

____
city state zip code

Mail to: Your Skin and How to Live in It
Box 22097
Cleveland, Ohio 44122